Post-Traumatic Stress Disorder in Children

The PROGRESS IN PSYCHIATRY Series

David Spiegel, M.D.
Series Editor

Post-Traumatic Stress Disorder in Children

Edited by
Spencer Eth, M.D.
Robert S. Pynoos, M.D., M.P.H.

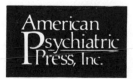

American Psychiatric Press, Inc.

1400 K Street, N.W.
Washington, DC 20005

Copyright © 1985 American Psychiatric Association
ALL RIGHTS RESERVED
Manufactured in the United States of America

The paper used in this publication meets the minimum requirements of American National Standard for Information Sciences—Permanence of Paper for Printed Library Materials, ANSI Z39.48-1984. ∞™

Library of Congress Cataloging in Publication Data
Main entry under title:

Post-traumatic stress disorder in children.

(The Progress in psychiatry series)
Chapters originally presented at the 137th Annual Meeting of the American Psychiatric Association in Los Angeles in May 1984.
Includes bibliographies.
1. Post-traumatic stress disorder in children—Congresses.
I. Eth, Spencer, 1950–   . II. Pynoos, Robert S.,
1947–   . III. American Psychiatric Association.
Meeting (137th: 1984: Los Angeles, Calif.) IV. Title:
Posttraumatic stress disorder in children. V. Series. [DNLM:
1. Stress Disorders, Post-Traumatic—in infancy &
childhood—congresses.
WS 350.6 P8576 1984]
RJ506.P55P67   1985   618.92'89   85-15762
ISBN 0-88048-067-X (alk. paper)

Contents

Contributors

William Arroyo, M.D.
Clinical Assistant Professor, Department of Psychiatry and Biobehavioral Sciences, University of Southern California

Elissa P. Benedek, M.D.
Director of Research and Training, Center for Forensic Psychiatry and Clinical Professor, University of Michigan Medical Center

Spencer Eth, M.D.
Clinical Director, Mental Health Clinic, Veterans Administration Medical Center, West Los Angeles; Assistant Professor of Psychiatry and Biobehavioral Sciences, University of California at Los Angeles School of Medicine; and Clinical Assistant Professor of Psychiatry and the Behavioral Sciences, University of Southern California School of Medicine

Calvin J. Frederick, Ph.D.
Chief, Psychology Service, Veterans Administration Medical Center, West Los Angeles; and Professor, Department of Psychiatry and Biobehavioral Sciences, University of California at Los Angeles

Jean Goodwin, M.D., M.P.H.
Professor, Department of Psychiatry, Medical College of Wisconsin

Arthur H. Green, M.D.
Director, Family Center, Presbyterian Hospital of the City of New York; and Associate Clinical Professor of Psychiatry, Division of Child Psychiatry, College of Physicians and Surgeons, Columbia University

Yehuda Nir, M.D.
Associate Clinical Professor in Psychiatry, Cornell Medical College; and Director, Pediatric Psychiatry, Memorial Sloan Kettering Cancer Center

Robert S. Pynoos, M.D., M.P.H.
Director, Program in Preventive Intervention in Trauma, Violence, and
    Bereavement in Childhood, Division of Child Psychiatry; and
    Assistant Professor of Psychiatry, Department of Psychiatry and
    Biobehavioral Sciences, University of California at Los Angeles
    School of Medicine

Lenore Cagen Terr, M.D.
Clinical Professor of Psychiatry, University of California San Francisco
    School of Medicine

Introduction to the Progress in Psychiatry Series

The *Progress in Psychiatry* Series is designed to capture in print the excitement that comes from assembling a diverse group of experts from various locations to examine in detail the newest information about a developing aspect of psychiatry. This series emerged as a collaboration between the American Psychiatric Association's Scientific Program Committee and the American Psychiatric Press, Inc. Great interest was generated by a number of the symposia presented each year at the APA Annual Meeting, and we realized that much of the information presented there, carefully assembled by people who are deeply immersed in a given area, would unfortunately not appear together in print. The symposia sessions at the Annual Meetings provide an unusual opportunity for experts who otherwise might not meet on the same platform to share their diverse viewpoints for a period of three hours. Some new themes are repeatedly reinforced and gain credence, while in other instances disagreements emerge, enabling the audience and now the reader to reach informed decisions about new directions in the field. The *Progress in Psychiatry* Series allows us to publish and capture some of the best of the symposia and thus provide an in-depth treatment of specific areas which might not otherwise be presented in broader review formats.

The symposia are selected on the basis of review by the Symposium Subcommittee of the Scientific Program Committee. From the approximately 80 symposia a year selected for presentation at the Annual Meeting, we choose approximately 10 percent which are deemed to be of especially high quality and to have interest to readers as well as meeting participants. After review by the American Psychiatric Press, we invite the authors to submit their papers as manuscripts for publication. We make every effort to expedite the publishing process so that books in the *Progress in Psychiatry* Series will be available as close as possible to the time of presentation at the Annual Meeting.

We believe the *Progress in Psychiatry* Series will provide you with an opportunity to review timely new information in specific fields of interest as they are developing. We hope you find that the excitement of the presentations is captured in the written word and that this book proves to be informative and enjoyable reading.

David Spiegel, M.D.
Series Editor
Progress in Psychiatry Series

Introduction

As the contributions to this book demonstrate, the investigation of post-traumatic stress disorder (PTSD) in childhood is an exciting new area of psychiatric inquiry. Although the concept of PTSD has been derived primarily from studies of traumatized adults, the most promising applications for preventive intervention may well be in responding to the mental health needs of children. Further, work with children provides a convenient opportunity to study the relationship of the acute and chronic phases of this disorder while deepening our understanding of developmental processes in general.

The inclusion of PTSD with its designated criteria as an Axis I diagnosis in the third edition of the *Diagnostic and Statistical Manual of Mental Disorders* (American Psychiatric Association 1980) has prompted an acceleration of research among adult victims of war, natural and human-induced disasters, and civilian violence. However, since the adoption of *DSM-III*, only a handful of psychiatrists have studied PTSD in children. The chapters of this book, originally presented at the 137th Annual Meeting of the American Psychiatric Association, held in Los Angeles in May 1984, assemble leading figures in this emerging field of child psychiatry. We hope this volume will encourage many more mental health professionals to join in furthering our scientific understanding of the often profound impact of traumatic occurrences on the lives of children. This work should be a high priority for all therapists, pediatricians, and school professionals because sensitivity to the prevalence, presentation, and serious consequences of PTSD in childhood is urgently needed to ensure early, proper recognition and treatment.

Elissa P. Benedek has long been an eloquent advocate for children. Her chapter presents the evolution of professional interest in trau-

matized children and outlines the progression of the level of observation, from exclusively indirect contacts with the parent or guardian
to direct involvement of the affected child in clinical interviews. She
places this book in its proper historical context as both a consolidation
of current thinking, and a major advance. She challenges psychiatrists
to move beyond naturalistic studies to begin formal, comparative
research of the disorder and treatment strategies. From her perspective as a forensic child psychiatrist, Dr. Benedek is in a unique position
to appreciate and comment upon the legal and societal implications
of this new field.

In our chapter on children exposed to acts of personal violence,
we outline the general theory of PTSD as it applies to the child
witness. This more-inclusive concept of trauma should alert the psychiatric community to a large and often neglected group of severely
affected children. We also bring particular concern to the effects of
violence, especially the violent injury or death of a parent. We discuss
common features found in the child witness, including the distressing
intrusion of violent or mutilating imagery, the challenge to the child's
own impulse control, the demanding task of assigning human accountability, and the potentially debilitating effects of unexplored
revenge fantasies. We also pay careful attention to issues specifically
related to the type of violence, its circumstances, and the intrapsychic
meaning attributed by the child. In contrast to most of the previously
reported studies, we have focused on elaborating the child's earliest
efforts at emotional and cognitive coping, hypothesizing that this
information will be critical to formulating developmentally sound
approaches to efforts at early intervention. The development over
several years of our specialized interview protocol illustrates the importance of clinical techniques that can elicit thorough and systematic
clinical data, while simultaneously offering the child relief from some
of the acute distress. Our research design, with its emphasis on the
most extreme cases of violence, represents only one possible approach. For us the *hammer effect* of examining catastrophic violence
permits clear visibility of salient phenomena, though it may obscure
observations of subtle child-intrinsic or environmental factors. Finally, in contrast to most other contributors to this volume, our work
has been conducted in collaboration over many years. We would
caution potential investigators and clinicians wishing to enter this
rewarding field of the heavy emotional demands which can burden
collaboration. Time and energy must be saved to assure adequate
emotional debriefing in the course of working with traumatized
children and their families.

Lenore C. Terr has pioneered the reawakening of interest in childhood trauma with her already classic study of the kidnapped children of Chowchilla. She has proved to be an exceptional phenomenologist, bringing a much-needed delineation of the childhood presentation of PTSD, especially with regard to the role of traumatic play, time distortions, and alteration of life attitude. Her chapter extends that work and serves as an important and timely reminder that psychic trauma frequently occurs in group situations. As she illustrates, the group may include siblings, schoolmates, and friends, as well as parents, guardians, and other adults (such as teachers or bus drivers). The importance of group psychology can significantly influence a child's experience of the trauma and its subsequent course. Group interactions can be manifested by shared distortions that specifically affect the anticipation of renewed threat and are the source of continued fears. Any consequent loss of group and community cohesion may adversely affect the child victim, whereas mutual support among group members can enhance recovery. Understanding these phenomena as they pertain to children will likely lead to new avenues of intervention involving school and community consultation. We have been reminded of the importance of group dynamics by our work in the last year with the student body and staff of a local elementary school, following a sniper attack on the school playground.

As former Chief of Disaster Assistance and Emergency Mental Health at the National Institute of Mental Health, Calvin J. Frederick has been instrumental in highlighting the public health dimension of the investigation and care of traumatized adults and children. As an investigator, Dr. Frederick has offered significant evidence for the different features and course of PTSD that can occur after violent and nonviolent incidents. He has also illuminated the significant behavioral consequences of traumatic reminders in the course of PTSD in children and adults. His emphasis on the need for thorough individual exploration with exposed children provided needed collateral evidence to support the value we ascribe to interviewing children immediately after a violent trauma. The study of the role of traumatic reminders and their relationship to renewed anxiety, suppression of thought, and avoidant behavior, especially as they operate in childhood, offers new possibilities of more specific behavioral and psychotherapeutic interventions. His chapter underscores the historical importance of work with survivors of large-scale natural and human-induced disasters, and offers a comprehensive program that extends from communitywide services to individual interventions.

Yehuda Nir has been one of the few directors of a division of child psychiatry at a major cancer center. Since the symposium, Dr. Nir has expressed surprise over the widespread interest generated by his paper. Therapists have responded as if their eyes have been opened to an unexpected application in pediatric consultation–liaison psychiatry. The recognition that PTSD in childhood can present as an iatrogenic response to traumatic cancer treatment represents a new dimension of psychiatric concern for medically ill children. The identification of this previously overlooked disorder in a group of seriously ill children will stimulate new techniques in the medical management of life-threatening illness. As medical treatment provides an increasing rate of cure, attention must be directed to the long-term mental health needs of these child survivors.

It was the psychological wounds of war that sparked the earliest interest of psychiatrists in what was to become the concept of PTSD. However, despite the World War II studies, of Freud and Burlingham in England, and Mercier and Despert in France, and the later reports from Northern Ireland and Israel, there have not been substantial research activities or large-scale programs to address the needs of the flood of psychological childhood casualties of worldwide war and civil unrest. With the vast immigration of families from Southeast Asia and Central America, American psychiatry must confront the special needs of these new residents. William Arroyo and Spencer Eth have conducted their work at a large urban medical center situated in an area densely populated by Central American refugees. Their study is a first step toward a conceptual model that identifies specific issues for future research and suggests new approaches to treatment. They outline the multiple and cumulative traumas inflicted by civil war, employing a model analogous to the one of massive psychic trauma found in concentration-camp victims. They argue that despite the wide spectrum of behavior initiating psychiatric referral, the common theme is the trauma the children experienced as victims of war. The evaluation and treatment is complicated by the complex interplay of multiple traumatic events superimposed on deprivation, malnutrition, family disruption, and immigration. Nonetheless, it is still possible to isolate singular traumatic incidents that require special attention. These unique trauma hold psychiatric priority in work with a child, such that by addressing them first a therapeutic alliance is forged and the subsequent treatment is facilitated.

A major figure in the study of child abuse, Arthur H. Green was the first to clearly identify the central traumatic elements in this common syndrome. Child abuse does not usually involve a discrete trauma, but rather a pattern of multiple beatings in a disturbed environment. However, Dr. Green has proposed that close exploration of incident-specific features can provide needed information about post-traumatic symptomatology critical to the care of the child. By exploring the effects on emerging personality, he suggests a treatment approach for these abused and disturbed children. Child abuse is violence perpetrated by a parent, and Dr. Green has brought an important research focus to the study of family dynamics, and the role of family therapy. He offers a model to describe the process of adaptation of a child to repeated traumas within the family. He proposes that specific post-traumatic effects contribute to the pathological attachment of the child to the abusive parent. The often-reported findings of a history of spousal or child abuse in the abusing parent's family of origin only confirms the need to appreciate the interplay of trauma and personality development. Only then can appropriate early interventions be devised to interrupt the cycle of violence.

Jean Goodwin presents a reassessment of the traumatic consequences of childhood incest experiences. Extrafamilial sexual abuse of children has clearly been associated with features comparable to those described in the adult rape-response syndrome. Dr. Goodwin contends that the intrafamilial molestation is also commonly followed by post-traumatic symptoms. Questions about the traumatic nature of incest have received much recent public and professional attention. Her case material and discussion reflect the controversy over the validity of retrospective adult reporting of childhood trauma and the need for careful elucidation of contemporaneous accounts.

Our concluding chapter on trauma and grief examines one aspect of the interaction of post-traumatic stress and other critical psychological processes. We think it introduces a new vista in our understanding of bereavement, and offers a modification of clinical practice in treating survivors of traumatic deaths. There has been a long-standing interest in psychiatry in the effects of parental loss in childhood. We urge that clinical research and treatment carefully consider the specific circumstance of the death and the child's degree of exposure. Our observations have indicated that with trauma mastery children exhibit a fuller range of responses and a less complicated resolution of grief.

The contributors to this volume are first-generation researchers who have focused on elucidating the childhood presentation of PTSD after a variety of traumatic occurrences. Some of us have now begun what might be considered the next generation of work by applying a more rigorous scientific design for data collection and hypothesis testing. Measuring the effects of degree of exposure by using well-constructed comparison groups will provide greater clarity about the specificity of post-traumatic stress disorder symptoms in childhood, as contrasted with other childhood symptoms, including other forms of anxiety, and symptoms of mood and conduct disturbances. In addition, more rigorous examination of mediating factors, both child-intrinsic and environmental, is needed in order to establish their influence on the course of recovery and responsiveness to therapeutic intervention. The use of reliable inventories of coping processes in children would allow for comparison of various types of trauma and illuminate the changing pattern of cognitive and emotional coping that appears to be the most effective.

A psychophysiological level of investigation may secure relevant information about persisting changes in the state of arousal following a single traumatic experience. These effects might include the onset of sleep disturbances, startle reactions, and the somatic symptoms that are so often associated with traumatic anxiety. The use of polysomnography could determine the nature of the sleep disturbance in childhood, including changes in REM-latency and stage-four sleep phenomena. Investigation of the acoustic startle reaction in children after auditory exposure could help delineate the location and endurance of any neurophysiological changes. Testing of cognitive discrimination capacity may help delineate children at risk after the trauma for overgeneralization of response to auditory and visual stimuli. This data could provide objective indicators of the disorder and recovery. Genetic, constitutional, and acquired characteristics may all be involved in determining the intensity and direction of these psychophysiological reactions.

We trust that the contributions included in this volume have demonstrated the recent gains in our knowledge of post-traumatic stress in childhood. The older literature, by neglecting early or direct contact with traumatized children, lost the invaluable opportunity for clinical insight. If there is one lesson we hope the readers of this volume will apply to their practice, it is an appreciation of the capacity of young children to explore their traumatic experiences, and the professional rewards of joining a child in this challenging task.

Robert S. Pynoos, M.D., M.P.H.
Spencer Eth, M.D.

REFERENCE

American Psychiatric Association: Diagnostic and Statistical Manual of Mental Disorders, 3rd ed. Washington, DC, American Psychiatric Association, 1980

Chapter 1

Children and Psychic Trauma: A Brief Review of Contemporary Thinking

Elissa P. Benedek, M.D.

Chapter 1

Children and Psychic Trauma: A Brief Review of Contemporary Thinking

Several years ago, I attended a professional meeting devoted to an in-depth discussion of victims of terrorism. As part of that meeting, an exceptionally talented researcher presented her findings in regard to a group of children who had been buried alive. She had interviewed the children shortly after their disaster. She had spent time with their families and friends. She presented meticulously observed, carefully collected, detailed historical and observational data of the psychiatric sequelae these children and their families experienced following a major psychic trauma/disaster. She elaborated on the short-term and long-term responses of these stressed children, in the process of presenting hypotheses about new defense mechanisms in children and post-traumatic stress in this group (Terr 1981; Terr 1983). Although the paper was exceptionally well done, and well presented, scholarly and fascinating, the reaction of the discussant and attending professionals was at first mocking, then openly hostile, and finally, after consideration, enlightening. The discussant, typically a mild-mannered, polite intellectual, was enraged. He questioned the researcher's technology, her findings, and then accused her of overpsychologizing and overdiagnosing. The attending group of professional mental health experts reinforced his denial of the effect of trauma and disaster on previously healthy children. The group became involved in a highly intellectualized discussion of the research methodology, the value of statistical tests, the importance of the researcher in clinical observation, and validity of data derived from interviewing children and their families. The validity of data obtained by listening to fantasies and observing play, age-old techniques for understanding children, was called into question as a research method. I puzzled for a long time over what was a distinctly uncommon response to a scientific paper by a group I knew well and had observed interacting previously. At first I thought the participants in the conference were not child psychiatrists, and thus did not understand play therapy and how observational data and research data about children could be derived from their play. Later, I thought, as the presenter was the only woman on the panel, perhaps some of the group's responses were directed toward her as a woman and a person, and they found it difficult to listen to "her." Finally, as I puzzled over this distinctly unusual response, with its characteristics of denial, hostility, anger, and incredulity, it seemed to me that I might be observing a phenomenon that is characteristic of the scientist/mental health professional's reaction to disaster and psychic trauma in children. It seemed to me that this meeting was but another form or manifestation of a long tradition of denying psychological and psychiatric sequelae in the child victim of trauma. The audience's response of disbelief, in the face of carefully collected documentation, might have been so intense because it was difficult for professionals to accept that traumatic events, caused by fellow humans, in the lives of children might color and shape their lives for years to come (Benedek 1984).

A review of the literature in regard to children, psychic trauma, and disaster supports the concept of clinician denial. Until recently (see Chapters 2 and 5), the subject of trauma, disaster, and psychological sequelae in children has only been examined cursorily. In fact, the *Diagnostic and Statistical Manual of Mental Disorders* (*DSM-III*, American Psychiatric Association 1980) has no special diagnostic criteria applicable to traumatized children. However, children are no strangers to traumatic stress and its sequelae. Over a significant span of human history they have been more often the victims of the slings and arrows of uncaring parents and society than the recipients of beneficent protection (Garmezy, in press).

Langmeier and Matejcek (1973), in their volume *Psychological Deprivation in Childhood*, describe four stages of progress in the search to understand the nature and consequences of trauma, psychic stress, and psychological sequelae in childhood. The first stage described by these authors has been entitled the *empirical*. It began in the last half of the 19th century and lasted through the first three decades of the 20th century. This stage was a period marked by unsystematized pediatric observations of children living in institutions, particularly orphanages and hospitals. The traumatized group were children who had lost their parents, primarily through death or abandonment. These children grieved and mourned their parents incompletely. The high instance of death among such youngsters and observations by scientists of the developmental and intellectual retardation in children who survived suggested that psychological factors might be important determiners of the developmental lags that characterized these children. Treatment interventions were not described. Stress was placed on the necessity of improving the underlying hygienic care of the children and the physical surroundings of the institutions caring for them. The importance of loss, grief, mourning, and psychic trauma, and their interconnections did not surface. During this period, no major disaster of a natural origin was well documented (Benedek, 1984).

The second period identified by these authors was roughly the period of the 1930s and 1940s, the period initiated by World War II. It was entitled the *alarm period*. The large numbers of deserted, displaced, and suffering children who wandered about Europe in the closing days of the war generated concern among both public and professionals over the mental, emotional, and physical development of these traumatized children. The trauma included years of suffering during imprisonment, attendant malnutrition, concentration-camp experiences, desertion, and loss of parents, friends, and families. Observers were alarmed and expected these children to be at severe psychological risk. In addition to these obvious traumatic stressors, mental health professionals were concerned about changes in the nuclear family and other great social changes occurring during this period. Such changes included such social stressors as growth in the number of working mothers, family breakups, and inadequate housing for young families.

Freud and Burlingham (1943) published anecdotal material about young children exposed to the ultimate disaster of World War II. Among other important *new* clinical observations noted by these astute observers was the importance of the parental reaction to trauma. They believed the psychological sense of well-being experienced by children in traumatic situations was directly correlated with parental sense of well-being. This early observation of the critical importance of parents' reaction to trauma in children pervades the literature and persists to this date. The belief that if parents remain cool, calm, and collected during psychic trauma, there will be no contagion, no panic, no fear, and no psychological sequelae on the part of children places an impossible burden on traumatized parents, perpetuates a myth of blaming parents for their natural reactions to stress, and holds them responsible for the reactions of their children. Solomon (1942) also reported on a sample of young children's reactions to blackouts and air raids during World War II. He noted that in general children responded to the threat of an imminent bombing attack with excitement. He also commented that children who handled blackouts in the most "calm, healthy fashion" had relationships with mean-ingful, stable, well-balanced persons who themselves "did not show anxiety."

Other observations were recorded, dealing with children's reaction to natural disasters. Block et al. (1956) studied children's emotional reactions to a tornado in Vicksburg, Mississippi. Of the 113 children examined, 56 showed emotional disturbances immediately after the tornado. Emotional disturbance was defined by Block and his col-leagues loosely as the presence of overt anxiety, anxiety equivalents, symptom formation, or intensification of previous pathological char-acter traits. However, even the children who were not described as showing serious emotional disturbance were described as irritable, sensitive, and phobic. These children made repeated attempts to play out a tornado game immediately after the disaster. Interestingly enough, Block, too, described a strong association between the parents who reported that they were confused and went to pieces and the most severely disturbed children. The most severely disturbed children showed regressive behavior such as enuresis, clinging to parents, and phobias of such things as outdoor activities and open-air movies. Friedman and Lynn (1957) reported the psychological reactions of children to the Andrea Doria disaster. Here, as an administrative and policy decision, women and children were rescued first. Children were frequently separated from their parents during attempts to rescue them. The policy of separation for the sake of rescue resulted in tragedy, isolation, and severe psychological consequences.

Spitz (1946) and Bowlby (1969, 1973, 1980) described new psy-chological constructs and scientific observations of traumatized chil-dren, and the terms *anaclitic depression, hospitalization, deprivation syndrome*, and *affection-less character* were the favored dynamic and theoretical formulations for children who were dysfunctional as the result of the trauma of deprivation and parental loss. Internal de-fensive structure, affect, and behavior of these children were not always meticulously observed, and not described comprehensively. The second important observation, again stemming from Anna Freud's (1943) work with children during World War II, is the critical importance of peers in the absence of parents and in preventing or ameliorating long-term psychological consequences, and perhaps even more generally, the importance of significant caring human rela-tionships subsequent to any disaster. Later authors have elaborated on or disputed Freud's earlier observations about the significance of this finding (Frederick 1981; also see Chapter 3).

The third period covers the 1950s, and was devoted to correcting and more critically appraising the preceding studies and the conclusions of the preceding era. It might be called a period of *synthesis*. The view that deprivation was inevitable in institutions and that deprivation and psychic consequences were always linked gave way to an enlarged conception of stress-resistant children. There was recognition that children are different biologically and temperamentally, that there are precursors which predispose some children to the devastating effects of trauma. That is, temperament, biological factors, experience within nuclear families, and prior experience with trauma might serve to protect some children from serious psychological consequences—or might also make a seemingly unimportant event disastrous (Krystal 1978). In addition, primary prevention and/ or therapeutic intervention could have significant impacts and alter the development of psychopathology.

The fourth stage can be described as one of experimental theoretical advances in which "there has been a marked intensification of a systematic research effort to study separation experiences, deprivation, and psychic trauma in a more organized fashion." Here, animal research has provided models for reactions to separation, deprivation, and disaster.

BEGINNING RESEARCH

This volume may be considered a part of the fourth period. It systematically investigates several new thematic areas in depth. The first theme investigated is one related to vulnerability and predisposition. In particular, Chapter 5 by Arroyo and Eth, *Children Traumatized by Central American Warfare*, addresses the multiple traumatic experiences that this particular group of children has survived, ranging from birth trauma, parental loss, poverty, violent death of friends and family, injury, to traumatic forced immigration. And yet, Arroyo and Eth say the war-traumatized child's prognosis may become more favorable with skilled, timely, and appropriate intervention, a note of optimism.

A second theme is also explored in depth in this volume: that is, the specific psychological reaction syndromes of children vis-à-vis adults at times of severe trauma. Terr, Eth, Pynoos, Goodwin, and Nir all have examined post-traumatic symptomatology in child victims. The trauma occurs independent of parental reactions. Their chapters range from a microscopic analysis (Terr, Chapter 3) to a macroscopic analysis (Goodwin, Chapter 8).

The third area explored in this volume are new potentiators or triggering factors. As the earlier reports focused on natural disaster such as famine, flood, cyclone, and tornado (Block 1956, Friedman 1957), this volume focuses more on human-induced disaster; victimization (rape, kidnapping, child abuse, incest); and observation of violence (homicide, suicide, rape).

The fourth set of factors we know least about to date, the protective and stress-resistant or resilient factors that assist and foster maintenance of competence during and subsequent to periods of psychic trauma, are briefly explored. Thus, this volume focuses mostly on etiology, description, and identification, and less on resiliency, coping, treatment, and research. Perhaps topics dealing with resiliency and coping will be the fifth area of exploration, or the charge for the 1980s and 1990s.

The second and most critical area of exploration, the recognition that children *do suffer* post-traumatic stress disorder, is implicit in all the chapters of this volume. The phenomena described in these children meet the *DSM-III* diagnostic criteria for post-traumatic stress disorder:

1. Existence of a recognizable stressor that would evoke significant symptoms of distress in almost anyone. It does not take a trained mental health clinician to recognize that war, natural disasters, malignancy, incest, kidnapping, and observation of suicide, homicide, or rape are recognizable stressors evoking distress in almost anyone. These are the stressors described in this volume. In fact, if a child patient denies distress after one of these experiences, one must wonder about the possibility of pathological denial.

2. Reexperiencing of the trauma as evident by at least one of the following: (*a*) recurrent and intrusive recollections of the event; (*b*) recurrent dreams of the event; (*c*) suddenly acting or feeling as if the traumatic event were reoccurring because of an association with an environmental or ideational stimulus. Although children do have recurrent nightmares in which there may be exact repetitions of the traumatic event or symbolic and actual attempts at mastery, children's recurrent and intrusive recollections are more like daydreams and fantasies. In addition, as primary-process thinking is so close to the surface in young children, environmental or ideational stimuli reminiscent or symbolic of the trauma may be directly responsible for behavioral changes. Children often are unable to link their changed affects, moods, thinking, and behavior to loud noises, darkness, or sudden visual or auditory stimuli which may "remind" them of the traumatic event, but an astute clinician can note the linking.

3. Numbing of responsiveness to or reduced involvement with the external world, beginning some time after the trauma, as shown by at least one of the following: markedly diminished interest in one or more significant activities, feelings of detachment or estrangement

from others, constricted affect. Information about this symptom can be obtained from children or from their friends, relatives, or caretakers. These symptoms have been described repeatedly (Freud and Burlingham 1974; Terr 1979; see also Chapters 2, 6, and 8). Emotional numbing may make children appear as if they are uninvolved or disinterested subsequent to trauma but, in fact, the numbing is defensive.

4. At least two of the following symptoms which were not present before the trauma: hyperalertness or exaggerated startle response, sleep disturbance, guilt about surviving when others have not or about behavior required for survival, memory impairment or trouble concentrating, avoidance of activities that arouse the recollection of the traumatic event, intensification of symptoms by exposure to events that symbolize or resemble the traumatic event. Particularly prominent in children are sleep disturbances, with inability to fall asleep, night terrors, and nightmares. Traumatized children are described as regressing in the following ways: climbing into bed with their parents, sleeping in strange places, sucking their thumbs, and becoming enuretic.

Terr (1979, 1981) reports some special criteria, while describing symptomatology following psychic trauma in children: (a) fear of death, separation, and further trauma; (b) misidentification of perpetrators and/or hallucinations of perpetrators; (c) no disavowal or traumatic amnesia; (d) absent vegetative and nervous effects. She also describes (1983) residual psychic phenomena, such as traumatic play, reenactment, personality changes, or chronic anxiety and fear of further trauma. Phobias may also appear for the first time as a reaction to the stressor.

TREATMENT CONSIDERATIONS

In Chapter 2, Pynoos and Eth have described the diagnostic interview with children who have experienced psychic trauma. The interview they elaborate has three distinct phases. The first engages the child, by having the child draw a picture and tell a story. This is a projective task, which provides a link to the child's intrusive concerns over issues of grief and trauma. A second phase, during which all the relevant issues are explored in depth, includes minute attention to the child's perceptual and affective experience. Finally, a closure phase, during which the child's present and future plans are reviewed. These authors stress that a thorough exploration of trauma offers a child immediate relief and causes no further distress.

Nir, in Chapter 6, supports their view that it is critical to intervene early with these high-risk children and families. He describes a potpourri of clinical interventions, including direct psychiatric contact with an at-risk child, social work counseling with a family, theme-centered group assistance to medical staff, and assistance to medical staff on understanding the dynamics of unusual behavior on the part of the affected child.

Frederick, in Chapter 4, adds to strategic planning with a list of treatment paradigms that extend treatment from the child and family to the community. The community he focuses on is both the trau-matized community and the caregivers, that is, the mental health workers and the disaster team. Unfortunately, although providing material regarding systems of care, none of the authors describe their exact interventions in any great detail. This material will be covered in a future publication (Pynoos and Eth, in press), but additional comments would be most helpful to practicing clinicians. It would be most useful to supplement these chapters with process notes and anecdotal material, which might clarify the specialized treatment process.

One other area not addressed in any detail in this volume is rarely explored in the literature. That is, the countertransference reactions of mental health personnel dealing with victims (Benedek 1984). Clinicians have long avoided the study of their own dynamics, which would lead to an understanding or elaboration of their difficult feel-ings about victims. Rather than furnishing an understanding of per-sonal reactions to victimization and countertransference problems, clinicians have often identified medical syndromes and collected sta-tistical data about child abuse, domestic violence, and now, post-traumatic stress. By simply identifying syndromes, it is possible not to confront one's own special feelings about the victims. Frederick (1971) has differentiated between the effects of natural and human-induced violence on caretakers. In natural disasters, friends, families, neighbors, and emergency teams get involved with victims both early and later, in the course of an event. There is community support, acceptance, and empathy for the victims of natural disasters. This is in contrast to human-induced disaster, such as terrorism, personal assault, rape, child abuse, or incest, where the notion of victim pre-cipitation has been common. That is to say, the victim's own actions have been seen as, in part, responsible for the violence perpetrated upon them. Clinicians working with victims of a natural disaster are perceived by the public and their colleagues as heroes. They put in long hours of ceaseless work and often feel euphoric because of the "good they have done" and the praise meted out by the media and the victims themselves. Emergency mental health workers in natural disasters are often described as seeing themselves as omnipotent.

They continue to work hard and intensely even when they are "burned out," and may have to be removed from the scene of a disaster because tiredness and irritability set in and judgment is impaired. In contrast, victims of human-induced violence rarely get emergency treatment, direct service, or skilled help. Their losses are personal, not property. Loss of self-esteem and sense of personal worth, value, and body integrity are not as dramatic as loss of home and property.

Individual clinicians, too, experience different reactions to victims of human-induced violence. Eth and Pynoos, in Chapter 2, note that even the experienced therapist may not ask about a traumatic event, feeling that rediscussion may be too traumatic for the child. In my experience, this is particularly true with young incest victims. I have heard numerous therapists explain why they have not asked a child about the significant event: "Why should I encourage such exhibitionism?" These therapists "forget" that retelling is equivalent to reworking, with a focus on understanding. The patient's question, Is is safe to talk to you? is answered with the countertransference reaction, It is not safe; I don't want to hear about it. The patient's helplessness is mirrored by the clinician's helplessness. The clinician, however, should know that retelling and replaying, with the effectual component, is one attempt at mastery of an experience (Benedek 1984).

The clinician's reaction, of course, is a function of the clinician's own developmental history, personal relating style, and coping skills. Despite variances in individual clinicians, everyone has conflicts around reaction to death, violence, and victimization. However, what seems to be most important is the clinician's sense of helplessness—If I am presented with this information, what can I do; what must I do? And so, there is a conspiracy of silence and the young victim is left to carry a burden alone.

LEGAL ISSUES

The role of PTSD syndromes in clinical practice and forensic evaluations is an issue of increasing theoretical and practical importance. Post-traumatic stress syndrome has appeared in the courtroom associated with Viet Nam veterans, criminal defendants, and adult victims of crime, particularly rape victims (Cavanaugh and Rogers 1983). To date, the case law on post-traumatic stress disorder is limited (Enlander 1983). It has, however, been raised at trial in most states now. As attorneys begin to understand and apply post-traumatic stress disorder to explain behavior, the number of reported cases in which it is a factor is likely to increase. The most dramatic and well-publicized application of PTSD in the courtroom is in the defense of criminal charges; defenses based on PTSD have been advanced in cases ranging from violent offenses, such as murder and attempted murder, to nonviolent crimes, such as drug conspiracy and tax fraud. In all probability, PTSD was raised by implication in the Buffalo Creek disaster. The disaster survivors received financial compensation for *psychic impairment*, a term which appears to be equivalent to post-traumatic stress (Newman 1976).

Burgess (1983) comments that the use of rape-trauma syndrome (a form of PTSD) in civil litigation cases is increasing, to validate the occurrence of psychological injuries subsequent to rape. According to Burgess, in reviewing 26 civil cases filed between 1979 and 1983 involving rape, 14 cases have been completed; six litigants (plaintiffs) received jury awards ranging from $15,000 to $800,000; of the settlements, three were settled after trial began and five settled before trial began, with amounts from $37,000 to $300,000. Terr (1981) discussed personal injury to children, and the civil suit that claims psychic trauma. She enumerates the three issues of import:

1. *(a)* Someone or something (the stressor) *(b)* is directly or indirectly at fault (liability), and *(c)* permanent emotional damage was done or there is probability of future emotional problems related to the accident/stressor (damages).
2. The emotional damage related to the stressor.
3. Can the party being sued pay? (collectibility).

We have recently been asked to evaluate child plaintiffs subjected to psychic trauma following death of a parent caused by medical malpractice. We have also evaluated children who demonstrated classic PTSD after being victims of incest, rape, or sodomy. In each of these cases, it was possible to make a diagnosis of post-traumatic stress syndrome, based on the *DSM-III* criteria and those criteria described earlier as particularly applicable to children. Although we do not have final data regarding awards for damages, the *DSM-III* criteria have been helpful in explaining child patient–plaintiff's psychological reactions and symptomatology to their families and their attorneys and finally to judges and juries, the trier-of-fact. We would suggest that the use of the *DSM-III* manual for such nonclinical purposes as determination of legal responsibility, or justification for payment of damages must be critically examined in each instance. The authors of *DSM-III* note that it was not designed for forensic use (American Psychiatric Press 1980) and that its use in forensic matter is questionable. Despite that caveat, it will continue to be used for legal purposes. Mental health professionals will most probably continue to provide expert testimony in criminal and civil cases. In particular, the mental health professional will be asked to define what is a stressor, whether a stressor is traumatic, what is the connection between the stressor and the symptomatology, and what role might preexisting symptomatology have played? The most difficult question to evaluate seems to be the question of the stressor being the legal proximate cause of the patient's psychic injury. Some clinicians feel that this question is not answerable clinically. That is, there may be a correlation, but not necessarily causation.

Although mental health experts may be qualified to determine whether symptoms exist and can be reasonably interpreted as PTSD, it must always be borne in mind by the clinician that the jury alone is responsible for assessing the nature of the trauma and credibility of the complainant (Rothman 1983). The requirement of a connection between traumatic stressor and PTSD symptoms creates a greater probability that testimony may duplicate the role of the jury than for other *DSM-III* diagnoses.

In forensic clinical evaluations, experts must meticulously document the complainant's history in his or her own words, and all the behavioral data. In the report to the court, experts should clearly recognize when they are making inferences and conclusory judgments, and should clearly identify such statements as inferential or judgmental. Only in this way can mental health professionals remain experts rather than advocates.

CONCLUSION

Pynoos, Eth, Garmezy, Benedek, and others who have worked in the area of psychic trauma all lament the fact there is no common research protocol used by investigators studying children at the time of disaster.

> At present as a field we have only information from isolated research groups studying varying types of disaster. Each has applied their own tools of investigation, often decided on after it has occurred. What is now needed is a major project to validate the diagnostic category of posttraumatic stress disorder in children, acute and chronic. This would require a multicentered research base with collaborators employing similar methods to obtain a uniform data base. (Source not provided by author)

Researchers also lament that funds may often become available only subsequent to a major disaster, and mobile teams trained to deal with such disasters are often delayed "while we process grant applications." The major traumas studied in depth (Terr, Eth, Pynoos) have all begun with small volunteer efforts. Organized psychiatry and child psychiatry have no team trained to deal with large-scale, human-induced disaster.

Although clinicians have long recognized that post-traumatic stress disorder can occur at any age, the description of this disorder in childhood has been limited. The disorder is clearly different, in many respects, in children (Eth and Pynoos 1985). We would hope that the revised *DSM-III* would contain a special section dealing with PTSD in children. It would appear that in children no preexisting phenomenology or psychiatric symptomatology need be necessary for this disorder to develop. It would also appear that the developmental immaturities of children lead to different diagnostic criteria and associated features. The course impairment and complications in children are distinguishable from those in adults. It is unclear to date how the type of trauma (human-induced or natural); the age and developmental level at which the trauma occurs (infancy, latency); the level of family and community support (chaotic or organized); and the treatment intervention (short-term or long-term, group or individual) play a role in the development and resolution of the disorder. It is clear, however, that more specific training and research in this area is critical. We predict the 1980s and 1990s will result in an exponential increase in our interest and knowledge of the manifestation of this disorder in childhood.

REFERENCES

American Psychiatric Association: Diagnostic and Statistical Manual of Mental Disorders, 3rd ed. Washington, DC, American Psychiatric Association, 1980

Benedek E: The silent scream: countertransference reactions to victims. American Journal of Social Psychiatry 4:49–52, 1984

Block D, Siber E, Perry S: Some factors in the emotional reaction of children to disaster. Am J Psychiatry 113:416–422, 1956

Bowlby J: Attachment and Loss: Attachment, vol. 1. New York, Basic Books, 1969

Bowlby J: Attachment and Loss: Separation Anxiety and Anger, vol 2. New York, Basic Books, 1973

Bowlby J: Attachment and Loss: Loss, Sadness, and Depression, vol 3. New York, Basic Books, 1980

Burgess AW: Rape trauma syndrome. Behavioral Science and the Law 1:85–97, 1983

Cavanaugh J, Rogers R: Editorial charter. Behavioral Science and the Law 1:3–5, 1983

Enlander PC: Post-traumatic stress disorder—Vietnam veterans and the law: a challenge to effective representation. Behavioral Science and the Law 1:25–51, 1983

Eth S, Pynoos R: Developmental perspective on psychic trauma in childhood, in Trauma and Its Wake. Edited by Figley CR. New York, Brunner/Mazel, 1985

Frederick CJ (ed): Aircraft Accidents: Emergency Mental Health Problems. DHHS Publications No. (ADM) 81-956, 1981

Freud A, Burlingham DT: War and Children. London, Medical War Books, 1943

Friedman P, Linn L: Some psychiatric notes on the Andrea Doria Disaster. Am J Psychiatry 14:426–432, 1957

Garmezy N: Stressors of childhood, in Stress, Coping, and Development in Childhood. New York, McGraw-Hill (in press)

Krystal H: Trauma and affect. Psychoanal Study Child 33:81–116, 1978

Langmeier J, Matejcek Z: Psychological Deprivation in Childhood. New York, Halsted Press, 1973

Moore H: Some emotional concomitants of disaster. Mental Hygiene 12:45–50, 1958

Newman CJ: Children of disaster: clinical observations at Buffalo Creek. Am J Psychiatry 133:306–312, 1976

Pynoos R, Eth S: Witness to violence: the child interview. J Am Acad Child Psychiatry (in press)

Rothman LJ: Problems of diagnoses and legal causation in courtroom use of post-traumatic stress disorder. Behavioral Science and the Law 1:128–129, 1983

Solomon J: Reactions of children to blackouts. Am J Neuropsychiatry 12:361–362, 1942

Spitz RA: Hospitalism: a follow-up report. Psychoanal Study Child 2:113–117, 1946

Terr L: Children of Chowchilla: a study of psychic trauma. Psychoanal Study Child 34:547–623, 1979

Terr L: 'Forbidden games': post-traumatic child's play. J Am Acad Child Psychiatry 20:741–760, 1981

Terr L: Chowchilla revisited: the effects of psychic trauma four years after a school-bus kidnapping. Am J Psychiatry 140:1543–1550, 1983

Chapter 2

Children Traumatized by Witnessing Acts of Personal Violence: Homicide, Rape, or Suicide Behavior

Robert S. Pynoos, M.D., M.P.H.
Spencer Eth, M.D.

Chapter 2

Children Traumatized by Witnessing Acts of Personal Violence: Homicide, Rape, or Suicide Behavior

Children who witness extreme acts of violence represent a population at significant risk of developing anxiety, depressive, phobic, conduct, and post-traumatic stress disorders, and are in need of both clinical and research attention. Our focus in this chapter is on the traumatic consequences for the child witness to any of three types of violence likely to have great personal impact on a child: the murder of a parent, the rape of a mother, and the suicidal act of a parent. The violent injury or death of a parent, in itself, imposes a severe stress on the child and serves as a psychic organizer profoundly altering the child's view of the world. We have found that the added burden of actually witnessing a portion of such an event will frequently produce an acute post-traumatic stress disorder in the child.

We will first review background data describing the extent of childhood exposure to violent acts in the United States, and discuss the psychological stresses on the child witness. We will then summarize our clinical observations of the children's responses: the immediate effect of the violence on the children, the early efforts at mastery, the resultant symptomatology or behavior, the issue of accountability, the influence of mediating factors on recovery, and the potential long-term consequences of the trauma.

Freud (1918) offered one of the first theories of psychic trauma. In doing so, he specifically called attention to the child witness. From adult retrospective reporting and reconstruction of childhood ex-

This chapter was supported by funds provided by the Robert E. Simon Foundation.

periences, he argued that young children, in observing parental intercourse, may experience a traumatic situation. The child assumes this is an act of violence, and feels helpless in the face of the danger to the mother. Because of the parents' lack of concern, Freud suggested, younger children are more likely to be exposed, and cannot escape the passive viewing.

The recent studies of psychic trauma in children have centered on those children who were victims of physical and sexual abuse or kidnapping. Terr (1983) and Green (1983) suggest that such direct victims of violence can suffer long-lasting ill effects. The conditions of these traumatized children resemble the post-traumatic stress disorder (PTSD) described in the third edition of the *Diagnostic and Statistical Manual of Mental Disorders* (*DSM-III*, American Psychiatric Association 1980), as validated by Horowitz et al. (1980) for traumatized adults; although Terr (1979) first reported differences in the childhood presentation that may require revised criteria. Nearly 80 percent of the over 100 uninjured child witnesses we studied also exhibited a characteristic pattern of PTSD.

Child witnesses to a parent's homicide, rape, or suicidal behavior demonstrate symptomatology fulfilling the four major *DSM-III* criteria for PTSD:

1. The perceived presence of a distressing, traumatic event; children will often describe it as so upsetting as never to be forgotten.

2. The reexperiencing of the occurrence; in young children this frequently takes the form of traumatic play and dreams, as well as intrusive images or sounds.

3. Psychic numbing or affective constriction; children may exhibit subdued or mute behavior, or commonly adopt an unemotional or third-person, nearly journalistic attitude toward the event.

4. Incident-specific phenomena that were previously not present; children are as likely as adults to suffer from startle reactions and avoidant behavior linked to trauma-specific reminders, and they may be especially susceptible to sleep disturbances (Frederick 1983). In addition, developmental factors affect the clinical picture and course of recovery, influencing the child's capacity to cope with the distress and to contend with traumatic anxiety (Eth and Pynoos 1984).

As recognized with adults, post-traumatic stress disorders are apparently more severe and longer lasting when a stressor is of "human design" (American Psychiatric Association 1980), especially in cases of human-induced violence (Frederick 1980). The PTSD symptoms in these child witnesses are likely to persist, and the children will benefit from prompt psychiatric assistance. We think our work with this group of children is of special importance because the psychological needs of the child witness are commonly neglected by the family, school, law enforcement agencies, and mental health profession.

EXPOSURE TO VIOLENCE

Within the past 20 years, the rate of violent crime in the United States has increased dramatically in relationship to other Western countries, reaching what may be deemed "an epidemic of violence" (West 1984). As of 1980, the reported number of homicides per year was 23,967 (Centers for Disease Control 1984), and the number of reported aggravated assaults exceeded 265,000. Of the homicides, approximately 40 percent were the result of domestic violence, and the vast majority of the victims were in the 20–39, child-rearing age group. The Sheriff's Homicide Division of Los Angeles County estimates that dependent children witness between 10 to 20 percent of the approximately 2,000 annual homicides in their jurisdiction. If a similar exposure rate applies to other urban areas, then several thousand children per year witness a murder, and, commonly, the victim is one of their parents.

Recent population surveys have drawn attention to the previously unappreciated extent of domestic violence in our society (Straus et al. 1980). Spouse beating and child abuse not only account for the largest number of direct victims, they also result in an even larger number of child witnesses (Pfouts et al. 1982). Early efforts to account for the intergenerational transmission of spouse beating and child abuse had focused primarily on childhood victims becoming adult perpetrators. However, the most comprehensive epidemiologic survey of marital aggression within a large sample of a general population (Kalmuss 1984) indicates that childhood witnessing of domestic violence is in fact the most significant predictor. The findings also suggest intergenerational transmission is role-specific rather than sex-specific. Kalmuss concludes that: "Observing one's father hitting one's mother increases the likelihood that sons will be victims as well as perpetrators, and that daughters will be perpetrators as well as victims of severe marital aggression" (p. 17).

In an examination of homicidally aggressive young children, Lewis et al. (1983, 151) found that the most significant factor contributing to violence is "to have a father who behaves violently, often homicidally." They also note that some of these children also appear at an increased risk of suicidal behavior. Although they specifically mention the importance of being a witness, unfortunately they do not designate which of the evaluated children fall into this category. However, they did conclude that "witnessing and being a victim of irrational violence engenders a kind of rage and frustration that, when directed inward, expresses itself as suicidal behavior. When directed outward and displaced from the father, it manifests itself as homicidal aggression" (p. 152).

In 1980, there were over 77,000 reported rapes outside of marriage in the United States (Centers for Disease Control 1984). In contrast to homicide, rape is seriously underreported. Recent household surveys indicate that, at a minimum, there is a 10:1 ratio of unreported to reported rapes, with an estimated actual annual incidence of approximately 800,000 rapes. As in cases of homicide, 40 percent of all rape victims are in the 20 to 39-year-old, child-bearing age group, and over 40 percent of all rapes occur in the home. If, estimating *conservatively*, a child is in the home when a rape occurs in one out of five instances, then as many as 25,000 children are exposed to this form of violence each year. In Los Angeles County alone, Sgt. Beth Dickerson (Chair, California Association of Sexual Assault Investigators) estimates that children are in the home when a rape occurs as much as 50 percent of the time and that the child (or children) directly view the assault in approximately 10 percent of the cases reported to the Sheriff's office.

In addition to rape outside of marriage, Russell (1982) has recently concluded, from a survey of households, that 14 percent of all married women in the United States report experiencing marital rape at least once in their lifetimes. Further, she found that in 11 percent of the cases in her survey one or more of the woman's children knew about or witnessed the attack(s). Given the high incidence of children present during the sexual assault of their mothers, the literature on rape and rape treatment is surprisingly silent on the subject (Silverman 1978; Burgess and Holmstrom 1979; Crenshaw 1979).

Suicide and suicidal behavior are also violent acts, and present a major source of childhood exposure to violence. There is evidence of an epidemic increase in the prevalence of suicide attempts in the United States as well as in other Western countries during the past two decades, though the rate of completed suicide has remained stationary (Weissman 1974). As with homicide and rape, the epidemiologic characteristics of attemptors put young children at a particularly high risk of exposure to the violent behavior. In 1980, there were 27,000 reported completed suicides in the United States (Centers for Disease Control 1984). Using the most conservative ratio of 8:1 attempts to completions, the Centers for Disease Control estimates that there were, at least, 216,000 attempts. Of these, 120,000 occurred in the 20 to 39-year-old age group, and accounted for 24,000 reported hospitalizations for suicide behavior. As Weissman concludes in her review of the epidemiology of suicide attempts, the annual incidence rates as derived from known studies suggest a far greater ratio of attempts to completed suicides than the 8:1 ratio projected in earlier studies. Indeed, in a 1964 door-to-door survey in the city of Los Angeles, Mintz concluded that 75,000 Los Angeles residents (or 3.9 percent of the city's population) had a history of attempted suicide. He, therefore, estimated there were 5,000,000 suicide attemptors in the United States at that time.

Older studies implied that suicide attempts were made by single individuals with no dependent children. More recent evidence reveals a notable increase in married women among the attemptors (Aitkins et al. 1969), and indicates that having children does not serve as a deterrent, as once believed (Kozak and Gibbs 1979). Weissman (1974) notes studies using general population comparisons now show a statistical excess of separated or divorced persons of both sexes among the attemptors. As she concludes, their high number is "consistent with clinical observations that attempts take place in the context of interpersonal disorganization and a breakdown of personal resources" (p. 740).

Given the increase in parental suicide behavior, the likelihood of a child witnessing this form of violence has, itself, probably increased dramatically in the past two decades, so that many thousands of children each year are directly or indirectly exposed to the suicide behavior of a parent. It is surprising, then, how little attention is made of this fact in the current discussion of the increasing rate of suicidal ideation and behavior in childhood. Those studies of childhood suicide behavior that do mention this risk factor (Shaffer and Fisher 1981; Pfeffer et al. 1983) do not, in particular, address the child witness. Nor do Cain and Fast (1972) discuss any specific consequences for the child witness in their classic report on the long-term effects on children when a parent commits suicide.

In summary, there is ample epidemiologic evidence to suggest that each year many thousands of children in the United States witness extreme acts of violence involving at least one of their parents.

THE TRAUMA OF THE CHILD WITNESS

Psychic trauma occurs when an individual is exposed to an overwhelming event and is rendered helpless in the face of intolerable danger, anxiety, or instinctual arousal. Freud (1926, 168) noted that, in a traumatic situation, "external and internal, real and instinctual dangers converge." There are a number of unique features that define traumatic witnessing and distinguish it from the trauma of direct victimization.

The helplessness of the child witness is determined by the passivity imposed by having to watch or listen to the sights and sounds surrounding the violence and the physical mutilation it creates. The uninjured child witness is unprotected from the full emotional impact of the violence, and may suffer immediately all of the painful symptoms of a post-traumatic stress disorder. In contrast, the injured child victim may immediately become self-absorbed with the pain or internally perceived impact of the physical damage. From that moment on, the child's set of memories may be much more involved with internal sensations; and the child's first preoccupation may focus on physical recovery. The different experiences of the uninjured and injured child participant may significantly influence the subsequent symptomatic constellations and their time course. This distinction may help to explain the vulnerability of the direct victim to the later development of dissociative symptoms and even multiple personality disorders (Putnam 1984), in contrast to the absence of such subsequent psychopathology in uninjured child witnesses.

Child witnesses do not display traumatic amnesia or disavowal. None of the children we interviewed indicated having felt any disbelief about the reality of what they witnessed. Instead, they seem similar to adult viewers of Lazarus et al.'s study (1965) who, knowing they were watching a real injurious accident, were unprotected from the full emotional impact of and physiological response to watching the event, in contrast to the controls, who were told it was staged or an intellectual exercise.

The perceived danger to the child witness does not depend on fear of self-harm, but on the personal meaning of the threat of the victim's injury or loss. The greater the personal impact on the child, the greater the likelihood a traumatic state will occur. Therefore, it is not surprising that child witnesses to parental homicide, rape, or suicidal behavior all report feeling emotionally overwhelmed by the danger to their parent.

Certainly, all of these children describe having had an enormously intense perceptual, affective, and physiological experience. Two major examples of persistent physiological changes are the high frequency of sleep disturbances, including night terrors and somnambulism, and startle reactions to specific perceptual traumatic reminders. Experimental evidence indicates that, in adults, unwelcome intrusive imagery and autonomic physiological reactions can persist after watching a disturbing event (Horowitz 1970; Kolb and Mutalipassi 1982). Our experience would suggest that these phenomena are common in children as well.

The intrusive imagery and associated affect may markedly interfere with the child's capacity to learn. As one child described, "I hear everything at school, and then it's gone because what I saw happen to my Mommy comes right back to me." Gardner (1971) has previously reported that the experience of violence can chronically diminish precise learning in children.

We have found four common psychological methods employed by children for limiting traumatic anxiety in the immediate weeks or months after an occurrence. By using *denial-in-fantasy* the child tries to mitigate painful reality by imaginatively reversing the outcome. By the *inhibition of spontaneous thought* the child works to avoid reminders of the event. In *fixation to the trauma*, evidenced by incomplete, usually unemotional, journalistic recountings of the event the child hopes to make the event more tolerable by means of reiteration. Finally, by becoming preoccupied with *fantasies of future harm* the child avoids directly addressing the actual trauma by supplanting the memories of the event with new fears. These strategies of emotional coping may persist or remit, only to reappear with traumatic reminders.

The child witness may be mentally involved with continued cognitive reappraisals of the action of all participants and witnesses. To offset his or her traumatic helplessness, the child must consider, if only in fantasy, alternate actions that could have prevented the occurrence, interrupted the violence before harm was done, reversed the physical harm, or gained safe retaliation. Developmental considerations are important determinants of these cognitive efforts (Eth and Pynoos 1984); and subsequent developmental maturity may bring about revisions.

Child witnesses differ from victims in their set of observations. They can monitor simultaneously the assailant, the victim, others at the scene, and their own activity as well. As a result, they may, more easily than victims, identify with or imagine themselves directly involved in the event in any of three roles: the assailant committing the violence, the victim being harmed, and a third person intervening. Important predisposing factors may be in operation. Specific psychodynamic issues may be especially at work. The choice may be influenced by being of the same sex as the parent-victim or assailant. On the other hand, for example, being seen as a special child of one parent may prove the more determining factor. Even in the initial interview, there may be evidence of the child's early identification; the particular choice may appear to be fixed or fluid, conflicted or readily adopted.

Inner plans of action (Lifton 1979) are most likely whenever activity has appeared ineffectual in a catastrophic situation (Lazarus 1966).

What is remarkable about the inner plans of action of the child witness is the dominance of fantasies of third-party intervention, either directly by the child or by another person. As a result of the child's fantasies of effective third-party intervention, the child may identify with the actions of the police, paramedics, or doctors to prevent violence or undo injuries, or with the judge, lawyers, and jailers to mete out punishment and revenge. The child may then develop new career interests that may entail a life of continued efforts to intervene successfully.

The descriptive account of post-traumatic stress disorders in *DSM-III* suggests that a more prolonged course can be expected if the stressor is of human design. As we have observed, struggles over assigning human accountability may add considerably to the child's traumatic burden after witnessing an extreme act of violence. Blame may be easy to assign, as in the case of a stranger assailant, or cause an intense conflict of loyalty, if a parent is to be held at fault. Intervention fantasies may also serve as a continuing source of self-blame for not having done more or of having been a coward. For the child witness, therefore, post-traumatic guilt is connected to imagined failures to intervene.

The fact of the violent occurrence, in itself, challenges the child's trust in adult restraint. Furthermore, it may prompt fantasies of revenge or an identification with the aggressor that can seriously jeopardize the child's confidence in his or her own impulse control. Uncharacteristic aggressive, reckless, or self-destructive behavior or prominent inhibitions may suddenly appear. Unconscious reenactment behavior may also endanger the child and others because it, too, may involve some repetition of violence.

Adult experimental studies (Feshbach 1955) have suggested that conscious aggressive fantasy expression after an insult, in contrast to nonexpression, reduces impulse tension and offers substitute goal satisfaction. However, the young child may need firm support to voice these frighteningly violent revenge fantasies, and, in doing so, may need assurances of safety against fantasies of retaliation.

Furthermore, because these children are preoccupied with the danger to the parent and with the need for intervention, they may not entertain a realistic appraisal of their own personal jeopardy. They may afterwards ignore, leave unacknowledged, or suppress any fear they might have experienced for their own safety. If their sense of fear is not adequately restored, they may be vulnerable to trauma-related dangerous situations, perhaps because of an inability or unwillingness to recognize a situation that requires personal protection.

On the other hand, there is an excitement that attends being witness to violence and danger. Thrilling situations, as characterized by Balint (1959, 23), all entail placing oneself in a dangerous situation that arouses fear. One is hopeful or confident that "the fear can be tolerated and mastered, the danger will pass, and that one will be able to return unharmed to safety." Child witnesses may be drawn to thrill seeking as one way to reassure themselves of their capacity to tolerate the shock of the traumatic occurrence. The popularity of extremely violent horror movies in part attests to the younger generation's preoccupation with the thrill of witnessing violence.

Finally, it is important to note that homicide, rape, and suicide behavior are not the collective violent acts of war, gang fights, or civil unrest, during which a general threat of harm may be perceived to be present. They are, instead, the isolated acts of individuals prompted by private motivations. Viewing such an event can cause profound changes in the child's sense of the safety and security of future intimate human relationships. As Terr (1983) notes, this change in future orientation may be one of the most significant markers of childhood trauma.

CLINICAL OBSERVATIONS

In this section we discuss our clinical observations of children who have witnessed a homicide, rape, or suicide attempt. Four key factors govern the onset and course of the child's post traumatic stress disorder. First, there is the phenomenology of PTSD, that is, those symptoms that unavoidably result from a traumatic state. Second, there are the child's early efforts to master the anxiety or avoid its renewal, including efforts to assure that the violence will not recur. Third, there are the many possible mediating influences that enhance or adversely affect trauma resolution. Fourth, there are the demands of trauma mastery, which may significantly influence current and future developmental tasks by hindering normal progression or prematurely propelling the child into more mature roles.

Special interview techniques, similar to one we have developed (Pynoos and Eth, in press), may be necessary to permit children to spontaneously and fully describe their subjective experiences. In addition to recalling the outstanding action and their own perceptual experiences, they can be assisted to recapture the worst moment, to identify details imbued with special meaning, to describe highly charged verbal exchanges, and to report ongoing traumatic reminders. It is possible to characterize the child's early cognitive and emotional coping strategies. Intervention studies of these procedures will be important because of the potential adverse long-term consequences of traumatic anxiety and a child's efforts to control it.

Homicide

It is hard to imagine a more harrowing experience than that of a child witnessing the murder of a parent. To date, we have evaluated over 50 such child witnesses, divided about equally in age among preschoolers, school children, and adolescents. Several Los Angeles agencies have served as subject referral sources, including the Police and Sheriff's Department, the District Attorney's Office, the Victim–Witness Assistance Program, and Child Protective Services. The homicides were the results of prolonged and brutal beatings, bloody stabbings, and massively disfiguring gunshot wounds. The assailants were identified as the other parent (35 percent), a friend or other relative (30 percent), or a stranger (35 percent).

We were able to conduct our initial interviews with the children within weeks of the event, and to follow them throughout the course of the acute traumatic response and subsequent criminal proceedings. All the children were haunted by the horrifying loss of impulse control in the assailant, the mutilation of the victim, and the helplessness of the victim and witness.

At the core of the child witness's trauma is the continued intrusion of the central violent action when physical harm was inflicted: the final blow with a fist, the plunge of a knife, or the blast of a shotgun. The child endures an intense perceptual experience. All sensory modalities are involved: the sight, sound, and smell of gunfire; the screams or sudden silence of the victim; the splash of blood and tissue on the child's clothes; the grasp of a dying parent; and the eventual police sirens. In addition, the child is aware of autonomic arousal and other bodily sensations. One young boy lamented, "It was awful, my heart hurt; it was beating so loud." The child may have been sharply attentive to a last, intense verbal exchange. One 13-year-old boy was haunted by the memory of his mother yelling at her estranged husband, "Go ahead, shoot me, show the kids what a big man you are." Special details may be imbued with traumatic meaning. One teenage daughter was preoccupied with the thought that her mother was wearing one of the teenager's dresses, borrowed that morning. Worst moments are not easily forgotten, as, for instance, when a dying father used a special nickname to call out to his young daughter.

Intrusion of traumatic references to the homicide is nearly universally present in projective drawings or storytelling tasks done within weeks of the event; and, as has been described in case reports, these references also directly appear in the child's play (Schetky 1978; Pruett 1979). In one such case (Bergen 1958), a 4-year-old girl whose mother was knifed to death carefully painted her hands red and acted out a game of being stabbed with a paint brush. School-age children may involve their schoolmates in their retelling or trauma-related games. One 7-year-old girl, who witnessed her father strangle her mother and then carry the body to the bedroom, forced all her friends to play the Mommy Game: "In the Mommy Game, you play dead, and I pick you up."

In order to mitigate the pain of the reality of the event the child may alter the fatal outcome in fantasy, while simultaneously giving an accurate description of what occurred. This process is often most apparent in the child's projective storytelling or traumatic play. One 7-year-old girl gave a careful description of her stuntman father's fatal shooting, while simultaneously drawing and telling the story of a clown who is saved by the sudden appearance of a net after being maliciously made to fall from a high wire. In this case, as in most others, the fantasied reversal of the violent outcome depends on outside intervention, thus highlighting the witness role. Addressing such denial-in-fantasy and its underlying meaning provides an important way to assist the child to be more sure of his or her capacity to cope with the intense affect associated with the violent death.

In homicide, there is little escape for the child witness from having to assign human responsibility for the loss of life. Human account-ability only adds to the child's anguish and difficulty in achieving trauma mastery. As one 12-year-old girl said, "I'm mad at the way she did go. Because that hurt. I just wanted her to die naturally, not die because someone shot her."

The child commonly experiences frightening fantasies or dreams of revenge as the only means to reverse feelings of helplessness, to adequately assign responsibility, and to place any further threat to rest. For example, the night after her mother was shot to death by an estranged boyfriend, one 11-year-old girl had the following dream: Her whole extended family is lined up in front as a firing squad, ready to execute the killer. She and her sister first knife him as he had once done to their mother. Then, while he stands, blindfold removed, her sister hands her a gun and she shoots him. Finally, she steps back and her relatives fire their rifles (Figure 1).

In therapeutic consultation, many children express particular relief at drawing or acting out their fantasy of punishment or revenge. Afterwards, we have often observed an increase in the child's overall affective expression, and only in retrospect to discern that a con-striction of affect had been present. However, the child needs help to distinguish these impulses from the murderous act of the assailant, since fear of these fantasies and impulses may possibly lead to un-

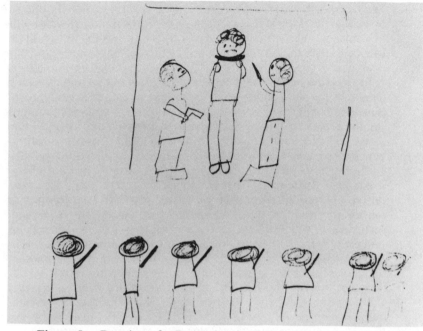

Figure 1.   Drawing of a Dream by an 11-Year-Old Girl Whose Mother
Was Shot to Death by an Estranged Boyfriend

recognized inhibitions in the child's life. One woman, who as a child
witnessed her mother's murder, continues to fear becoming rich
because she might use all her money to hire a "hit man" to assassinate
the killer.

Any of the child's convictions about the safety of interpersonal
relationships may be shattered. Children have described having afterwards envisioned the need to live alone in an impenetrable fortress
when they grow up. Other children have stated that they would never
marry for fear that a marital argument would once again be fatal.

Since the judicial proceedings adjudicate blame, there is a necessary
link between judicial outcome and trauma resolution (Pynoos and
Eth 1984). If, for example, an arrest is not made, the child may never
achieve psychological closure. One seven-year-old boy saw his father
stabbed by a stranger who was never apprehended. Years later, he
continues to fear for his own life, carries a switch-blade, and seeks
to avenge his father's murder.

A parent's murder precipitates an irreversible upheaval in the child's life. As Barkas (1978) describes, family and friends undergo a prolonged period of suffering. During this interval, the surviving parent may be in a traumatized and grief-stricken state, and emotionally unavailable to aid the child. In parent-parent homicide, the child can lose both parents, one by death and the other by incarceration. The child may be uprooted to live with relatives and may have to change schools. They may not only have to contend with their own intensely ambivalent feelings toward the homicidal parent, but also the embittered and revengeful feelings of the deceased parent's family of origin. Even among the deceased parent's family members there may be an implicit prohibition against any reference to the violent death (Lister 1982). Finally, they must endure the rigors of the legal proceedings that follow a homicide (Pynoos and Eth 1984).

All these additional, externally imposed stresses hinder the child's recovery from the initial traumatic impact of the homicide. Yet, as one assists the child to feel more efficacious in addressing the traumatic event, an enhanced sense of competence in facing difficult, immediate life tasks may also be exhibited. One of the most important of these is grief work, and we report elsewhere in this monograph on the interaction of grief and trauma.

Rape

We have begun to interview a number of children soon after they have endured the profoundly frightening experience of witnessing the rape of their mothers. Local rape-response centers, rape hotlines, and law enforcement agencies are the source of referrals. The incidents, all out-of-marriage occurrences, have included attempted sexual assaults, forced penetrations, and oral copulation. In a number of the cases, the rapist entered or left the home through the child's bedroom window. The rapist also frequently threatened harm to the child if the woman were to resist, and voiced this threat with the child present. The following case history points out the potential for trauma to the child who is present in the home when a rape occurs.

A known rapist broke into a single parent's house through her six-year-old son's bedroom window and raped her for the next two and one-half hours (Wells 1978). Early in the attack, which took place primarily in the mother's bedroom, her son came to the bedroom door. The rapist ordered the mother to yell at her son, "If you don't shut up I'll beat your brains out!" The mother had never spoken to her child that way. With a knife at her throat, the rapist ordered her to do so, threatening to kill the boy if she refused. She complied. The boy was visibly upset by her foreign, abusive tone of voice.

Later, towards the end of the assault, the man took the mother to her son's open bedroom, where he said things like, "It was a good fuck, wasn't it?"

Once the rapist had left, the mother went to her son, told him she had been hurt, and ran with him, screaming, into the street. Rousing her neighbors, she ordered them to take her child back home while she called the police. When the police arrived, the mother could not stay with her son but asked the police officers to sit with him. Later, she called her ex-husband to come and take the child.

It is hard to imagine that the child was not affected by his mother's abusive language toward him, the sounds and sights of the attack, the rapist's comments at his bedroom door, the experience of being suddenly carried into the street by his screaming mother, the forced separation from his mother at the time of the crisis, as well as the general turmoil and emotional upheaval immediately following the rape. And, indeed, in the acute aftermath of the attack the young boy suffered from a sleep disturbance, nightmares, a decline in school performance, and sudden, previously unseen aggressive behavior with his schoolmates.

In other cases, children have described to us how continuously intrusive the image of the attack on their parent remained. One eight-year-old girl said, "I keep seeing him in my mind going at my mother in the hallway." The same girl also pointed out the extra burden of the witness role, telling us that if she'd been at a friend's and heard of what had occurred she would still have been afraid, but "it would not have been as scary as seeing his face and what he did." For months afterwards, this little girl felt nauseated whenever she thought of the assault. She, too, couldn't sleep at night, and dreamt repeatedly of someone again breaking into the house.

Rape is an act that consists of both sexual and aggressive abuse. In each case we have seen, the child witness tended almost immediately to repress the sexual aspects of the attack, while appearing consciously preoccupied with the violence and the mother's vulnerability to harm. However, the traumatic play of these same children often took the form of repeated self-stimulation. While one five-year-old boy, who had witnessed the rapist's use of a dildo, talked of the break-in and the knife held at his mother's throat, he simultaneously continued to rub up and down on a toy baseball bat that he had carried to the interview.

The central action of the assault may be cognitively confusing to the child witness. As a result, the child may have great difficulty in processing the event; and the intermixing of reality and age-appropriate fantasy may intensify the child's worries. For example, the boy just mentioned was confused by witnessing the use of a dildo. In addition to carrying the toy bat to his interview, his first play sequence was of having a finger come on and off his hand. When he became more comfortable speaking, he then expressed his continued fear that his penis could become free from his body.

Because discussion of the sexual component of the act may be subject to much more social and family taboo than the elements of violence, such cognitive confusions may never be adequately addressed with the child. We have further observed that it is not necessarily the child who shies away from explicit references to the sexual behavior but often it is the interviewer. In the case of the boy with the bat, the interviewer had declined to name the dildo or address its use, only to find out in the follow-up family interview that the child had become precociously aware of many of the sexually explicit terms for what occurred.

Viewing the rape of one's mother can profoundly affect the child's sense of security and vulnerability to being physically violated. Even young children can understand the crime involves a lack of sexual consent. One little girl explained a rape is when a woman doesn't want to get pregnant and a man uses force to make her pregnant anyway. The child may well reason that if a grown woman, especially a parent, can be violated against her will, then the child may be that much more vulnerable. All the children fear someone again breaking into their home, and want measures taken to ensure safety. In one case, a seven-year-old girl wanted to move back to her former home next to the house of a policeman. This same girl stayed awake each night until the hour of the attack had passed.

Rape may come to represent a threat of attack that can occur unexpectedly at any time in the future. Children's future orientation may be altered to include a delayed fear of recurrence when they become an adult. One eight-year-old girl said that at present she was not worried, but that when she grew up she would be afraid someone might rape her in the street and "put his hand over my mouth." She insisted that she would always have a roommate until she married and would never feel safe to be alone.

Gender identification and sexual role differences are apparent in the child's reactions to witnessing rape. Young girls are terrified by the role identification with the mother as victim. They may have repeated dreams of being under attack, and become frightened of strangers or the neighborhood in general. Boys, too, may feel more vulnerable to being violated. However, several of the boys we have interviewed noticeably identified with the rapists, rather than their helpless mothers. In their play, and occasionally in their dreams, they became the male attacker. However, these boys were visibly fright-ened by the implication of pretending to be the assailant. Although, perhaps, the most expeditious way of handling their traumatic help-lessness, these boys required help to understand the traumatic nature of their response.

Children of both sexes may also feel painfully guilty, frustrated, or angry because they were unable to stop the rape. This feeling of responsibility may be especially difficult for them to bear if they feel that it was only the threat of harm to them that forced their mother to cooperate. Therapeutic attention toward the traumatic helplessness and passivity, including playacting at how they would have wished to intervene, can diminish their guilt.

The post-rape family milieu is typically an anxious environment. Many mediating factors may adversely influence the child's ability to cope with his or her traumatic experience. The severely traumatized mother must proceed through a difficult course of recovery that can have many phases (Burgess and Holmstrom 1979). Because of her own psychological agenda, the mother may not be readily available to assist her child and, early on, may feel incapable of that emotional challenge. In several of our cases, the mother was struggling to accept her own need for help. In one such case, a mother poignantly de-scribed how guilty she felt at the thought of her child being trau-matized, as if she were responsible for the child witnessing her rape. This mother could face her child's subsequent difficulties only after she, herself, received some counseling.

The child's efforts at mastery may be linked to the mother's in other ways. Several children we interviewed describe their unwill-ingness to speak openly at home of their experience because they feared causing recurrent anxiety in their mothers. Children also found it very hard to quiet their own subsequent fears as long as their mothers remained anxious, and afraid of men. Several mothers de-scribed having severe startle reactions whenever their husbands or sons unexpectedly came into a room. In one case, the mother on several occasions awoke yelling when her son came into her bedroom in the middle of the night looking for comfort.

The child's ability to master the trauma may be gravely compro-mised by estrangement or conflicts between the mother and her husband, live-in partner, or boyfriend. Beneke (1982) and Crenshaw (1979) estimate that the rape-precipitated stresses on both partners result in the permanent dissolution of the relationship in over half the cases. Whether or not the adult partners remain together, a "ripple effect" of familial disturbance occurs as the rape of the mother creates repercussions for other family members (Burgess and Holmstrom

1979). Tension, overprotection, rage, revenge seeking, and avoidance of the spouse are all typical reactions following a sexual assault, and all affect the children within the family unit.

The responses may also have traumatic etiology in the circumstances of the rape. In two cases we studied, the husband, tied up or restrained, was present during the attack and forced to watch under the threat of violence. Afterwards, the father and mother experienced a severe sense of estrangement from each other. The child, too, found it extremely difficult to tolerate the father's helplessness and ineffectualness. In one case, the child avoided showing any affection toward her father, and refused his efforts to comfort her. However, after therapeutic consultation, one of the girl's first spontaneous acts was to embrace her father, and, in doing so, actually help begin to restore a sense of family unity.

Suicide

Nothing, perhaps, is more disillusioning to a child than becoming aware of a parent's attempted suicide or death by suicide. No other single parental act can so painfully accentuate issues of human accountability, the control of one's destructive impulses, or the child's dependence and helplessness. Frequently, the child is involved unwittingly in some aspect of the parent's suicidal behavior. The parent may merely make specific plans to have the child elsewhere or may cause the child to be a witness to some portion of the event, usually the discovery of the parent afterwards.

Several years ago, one of the authors and two other colleagues (Pynoos et al. 1981) studied the responses of 30 children whose parents had recently made a first-known suicide attempt. Few of these attempts could be considered gestures; without timely intervention many would have resulted in death, and all of the parents were hospitalized. The children were interviewed within two weeks of the occurrence, during the parent's psychiatric hospitalization. In the majority of cases the children alone had discovered the parent or were in the company of other family members who did so. They had viewed the comatose or bleeding parent, and retained painful, intrusive recollections of the sight.

The children displayed typical traumatic responses: overwhelming affect; continued reenactment in play and behavior; identification of certain details of the suicidal behavior as having special traumatic meaning; cognitively disruptive intrusive thoughts, and efforts at denial-in-fantasy; and behavior and fantasy aimed at reducing the threat of recurrence.

In general, the parents attempted to hide the suicidal nature of the behavior from the child. For example, violent attempts typically were covered over by stories of accidents or medical emergencies, even when the child had witnessed enough to know otherwise. The children, too, knew and understood much more than they were willing to admit to their parents.

No doubt the parent–child relationship may already have been disturbed, and the child exposed to a depressive or impulse-ridden environment. However, the impact of the parent's actual suicide attempt is unique for its profound, long-term alteration of the parent–child relationship. The fact that the injured parent is the active agent distinguishes this situation not only from homicide or rape, but also from one in which the parent has become physically ill. The self-directed nature of parental suicidal behavior forms the core of the child's trauma and hinders the child's efforts to assimilate the event.

The children were frightened and angered to think a parent would abandon their care, the spouses were angry that the other parent would resort to this behavior, and the suicide attemptors, themselves, often felt their act confirmed their failure as parents. Although the explanations of "accidental" behavior muffled the overt conflict over accountability, the children nevertheless still viewed the parent as responsible. Some children, for instance, declared that their mother or father could have been more careful. Other children desperately tried to remove responsibility from the suicidal parent and redirect blame towards themselves, their other parent, or someone else.

The following case illustrates the nature of the trauma. We interviewed an affable, courageous, yet sad eight-year-old boy one week after his mother had cut her forearms and wrists with a razor blade. He described how his parents had fought that morning and how his father had stormed off to work. Later, his mother sent him off to buy razor blades so, he was told, they could make papier-mâché objects. He was looking forward to this special activity. However, when he returned he was once again sent to the grocery store. When he came home the second time, he discovered his mother in her bedroom with blood covering her arms and face. On seeing her he quickly realized the injuries were self-inflicted. During the interview the boy reported having felt "real mad," and immediately wanting "to pack his belongings and leave." He set the first of his drawings at the moment when he decided, instead, to go next door for help. Initially, he thought she had cut herself with scissors. However, at what he called the worst moment for him, he found a razor blade under her arm. Poignantly and with his eyes filled with tears, he told the interviewer, "mostly I like to help my mother, but I felt really hurt by her when I found out what she wanted the razor blades for.

. . . Just like she used me!" he exclaimed. "I thought we were going to have fun, like we hadn't had in a long time." He then cried and cried.

This child, like many others we interviewed, insisted on drawing a picture of his mutilated parent. With assistance, he discussed the persistent intrusive images of her bloody injuries. The more violent or physically damaging the parent's act, the more uncamouflaged and overtly intrusive the traumatic theme of the child's drawings. Another eight-year-old boy chose to draw a picture of his violently mutilated father, who had cut himself at the neck, ankles, and wrists. In addition to drawing the heavily bandaged forearms, the child pencilled in the scraggly beard that the father was growing to cover the disfiguring scar on his neck (Figure 2).

One of the most serious traumatic consequences for these children appears to be the unconscious reenactments and the imitation in play of the parents' suicidal behavior. The father of one seven-year-old boy had taken a nearly lethal overdose and, as a consequence, was left with serious neurological impairments. Within a week of the attempt, the boy began to ask his mother what would happen if he were to take 10 pills, or 8, or 6. How many would he need to kill himself, he asked. Another child was observed stabbing himself with a rubber play knife. Although some of these children may have been depressed or harbored suicidal thoughts before the parent's suicide attempt, the repetitive traumatic content of their play and reenactments was obvious.

More than either homicide or rape, parental suicide behavior, as a trauma, ensnares the child in a state of psychological preparedness aimed at offsetting traumatic helplessness by preventing further harm. We found that even preschoolers understand prevention requires the control of the parent's behavior. One can observe these children's attempts, in fact and in fantasy, to ensure their own security and their parents' welfare by protecting the parent. These attempts result in what we have termed the *psychological capture* of the child, as the child prepares to live with a parent known to have attempted to take his or her life.

The children do not conceive of their task as simply a matter of being on good behavior or always looking to help the parent to feel better. They imagine far more specific third-party interventions, typical of traumatized witnesses. One eight-year-old child, who had discovered his mother comatose with the empty pill bottles next to her, spontaneously asked the interviewer, "If I hide my mother's pills in my knapsack, do you think she'd find them there?" Another seven-year-old boy, when asked about his love of baseball, responded that

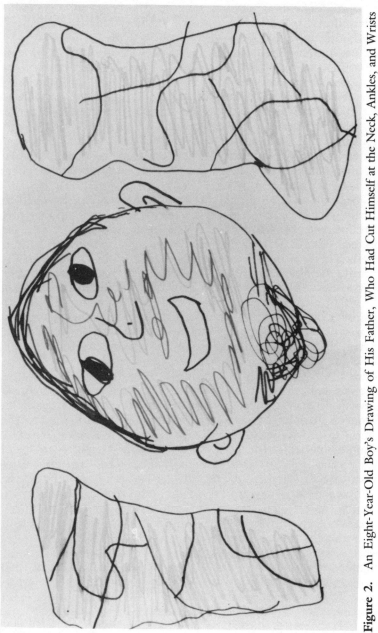

Figure 2. An Eight-Year-Old Boy's Drawing of His Father, Who Had Cut Himself at the Neck, Ankles, and Wrists

he would only go to play a game if he could make sure his mother sits in the front row where she would never be out of his sight.

Although the suicidal parent generally avoids the confrontation, the child often finds it imperative to gain a guarantee of safety by exhorting the parent to promise never again to repeat the behavior. "Promise me you won't ever take any pills anymore!" exclaimed one boy to his mother. "Don't do it again," he continued, "Not just with pills, but not by jumping out of the window, or throwing yourself into the river either."

Because the threat is perceived as ongoing, closure or recovery is therefore difficult for the child to achieve. Most often, the post-traumatic milieu includes a conspiracy of silence and/or misleading explanations to deny the suicidal intent of the act. One eight-year-old boy, who saw his father in a pool of blood after a violent throat slashing, was told his father had a shaving accident. Such a misleading explanation interferes with efforts at trauma mastery, and fails to protect the child from the traumatic consequences we have described. Furthermore, misleading explanations and conspiracy of silence can contribute to chronic difficulties in learning and cognition, as described by Cain and Fast (1972), or to an inability to accurately identify one's emotional responses (Bowlby 1979).

Inadequate or misleading discussion of the occurrence also increases the child witness's vulnerability to self-blame for the initial occurrence and any subsequent parental suicide behavior, because the child's inner plans of third-party intervention will also go unaddressed. Studies of children's responses even years after a completed parental suicide have indicated the severe degree of guilt in the child survivor. In discovering the parent, the child witnesses (in a concrete manner) may implicate themselves in the fatal outcome. We have interviewed one hospitalized adult patient who, as a 14-year-old, had found his dead mother. He had silently maintained the conviction that his mother had actually died as a result of his having cut her down from the rope by which she had hung herself.

Finally, there may be life-long risks as a result of the childhood trauma. The majority of the suicidal parents were diagnosed as having a major affective disorder. The children, therefore, represent a high-risk group for depression. Feelings of self-blame for their parents' behavior may contribute to their depressive self-accusations. These children may be additionally vulnerable to suicidal behavior because the potentially fatal nature of the behavior may not be fully appreciated. Even as adults, they may reevoke childhood fantasies of third-party intervention, or "rescue fantasies," that prove unrealistic to the situation.

CONCLUSION

These are all children who had to experience something that no child should have to endure. We hope we have interested the reader in becoming familiar with the nature of the child witnesses' distress. Their current and future lives, as we have described, will be colored by this singular traumatic occurrence and the series of events in its aftermath. As Baudry notes (1983), Freud emphasized in one of his later papers (1937,75) how efforts to overcome trauma can play a significant role in shaping character and how the trauma "may be taken up into what passes as normal ego" and "becomes a permanent trend in it." The permanent marks on these child witnesses should not be easily dismissed.

As we discovered when we began these studies, these children have rarely had the opportunity to voice their private feelings; most often, professionals and families alike have been hesitant to discuss the event with children out of fear of further traumatizing them. We have been taught, by the children's own courage, to join with them in a thorough exploration of their subjective experience, to address their feelings of self-blame, and to underscore their helplessness and realistic fears (Pynoos and Eth, in press). Children are open to these interventions; the psychiatrist who assists the young witness to violence will be rewarded by the child's gratitude.

REFERENCES

Aitkins R, Buglass D, Kreitman NJ: The changing pattern of attempted suicide in Edinburgh, 1962–67. British Journal of Preventive Social Medicine 23:111–115, 1969

American Psychiatric Association: Diagnostic and Statistical Manual of Mental Disorders, 3rd ed. Washington, DC, American Psychiatric Association, 1980

Balint M: Thrills and Regression. New York, International Universities Press, 1959

Barkas JL: Victims. London, Peel Press, 1978

Baudry R: The evolution of the concept of character in Freud's writings. J Am Psychoanal Assoc 31:3–32, 1983

Beneke T: Men on Rape. New York, St Martin's Press, 1982

Bergen M: Effect of severe trauma on a 4-year-old child. Psychoanal Study Child 13:407–429, 1958

Bowlby J: On knowing what you aren't supposed to know and feeling what you are not supposed to feel. Can J Psychiatry 24:403–408, 1979

Burgess AW, Holmstrom LL: Rape: Crisis and Recovery. Bowie, Md, Robert J Brady Co, 1979

Cain A, Fast I: Children's disturbed reactions to parent suicide: distortion and guilt, communication and identification, in Survivors of Suicide. Edited by Cain A. Springfield, Ill, Charles C Thomas, 1972

Centers for Disease Control: Violent crime: Summary of morbidity. Atlanta, Violence Epidemiology Branch, 1984

Crenshaw T: Counseling of family and friends, in Rape: Helping the Victim. Edited by Halpern S. Medical Economic Company, 1979

Eth S, Pynoos R: Children who witness the homicide of a parent. Paper presented at the annual meeting of the American Psychiatric Association, New York, May 1983

Eth S, Pynoos R: Developmental perspectives on psychic trauma in childhood, in Trauma and Its Wake. Edited by Figley CR. New York, Brunner/Mazel, 1984

Feshbach S: The drive-reducing function of fantasy behavior. Journal of Abnormal and Social Psychology 50:3–11, 1955

Frederick C: Effects of natural versus human-induced violence upon victims. Evaluation and Change, Special Issue: 71–75, 1980

Frederick C: Violence and disasters: immediate and long-term consequences, in Helping Victims of Violence. Edited by Ministry of Welfare and Cultural Affairs. The Hague, Government Publishing Office, 1983

Freud S: From the history of an infantile neurosis, in The Standard Edition of the Complete Psychological Works of Sigmund Freud, vol. 17. Edited by James Strachey. London, Hogarth Press, 1918

Freud S: Inhibitions, symptoms and anxiety, in The Standard Edition of the Complete Psychological Works of Sigmund Freud, vol 20. Edited by James Strachey. London, Hogarth Press, 1926

Freud, S: Moses and monotheism, in The Standard Edition of the Complete Psychological Works of Sigmund Freud, vol 23. Edited by James Strachey. London, Hogarth Press, 1937

Gardner GR: Aggression and violence—the enemies of precision learning in children. Am J Psychiatry 128:445–450, 1971

Green A: Dimensions of psychological trauma in abused children. J Am Acad Child Psychiatry 22:231–237, 1983

Horowitz MJ: Image Formation and Cognition. New York, Appleton-Century-Crofts, 1970

Horowitz MJ, Wilner M, Kultreider N, et al: Signs and symptoms of post-traumatic stress disorder. Arch Gen Psychiatry 37:85–92, 1980

Kalmuss D: The intergenerational transmission of marital aggression. Journal of Marriage and the Family 46:11–19, 1984

Kolb L, Mutalipassi L: The conditioned emotional response: a subclass of the chronic and delayed post-traumatic stress disorder. Psychiatric Annals 12:979–987, 1982

Kozak CM, Gibbs J: Dependent children and suicide of married parents. Suicide Life Threat Behav 9:67–75, 1979

Lazarus RS: Psychological Stress and the Coping Process. New York, McGraw-Hill, 1966

Lazarus RS, Opton EM Jr, Nomikos MS, et al: The principle of short-circuiting of threat: further evidence. J Pers 33:622–635, 1965

Lewis DO, Shanok SS, Grant M, et al: Homicidally aggressive young children: neuropsychiatric and experiential correlates. Am J Psychiatry 140:148–153, 1983

Lifton RJ: The Broken Connection. New York, Simon and Schuster, 1979

Lister ED: Forced silence: a neglected dimension of trauma. Am J Psychiatry 139:867–872, 1982

Mintz R: Prevalence of persons in the city of Los Angeles who have attempted suicide: a pilot study. Bulletin of Suicidology 7:9–16, 1970

Pfeffer C, Plutchik R, Mizruchi MS: Suicidal and assaultive behavior in children: classification, measurement, and interrelations. Am J Psychiatry 140:154–157, 1983

Pfouts J, Schopler J, Henley HC: Forgotten victims of family violence. Social Work 27:367–368, 1982

Pruett KR: Home treatment for two infants who witnessed their mother's murder. J Am Acad Child Psychiatry 18:647–657, 1979

Putnam FW, Post RM, Guroff JJ, et al: One hundred cases of multiple personality disorder. Presented at the annual meeting of the American Psychiatric Association, Los Angeles, May 1984

Pynoos R, Eth S: The child as witness to homicide. Journal of Social Issues 40:269–290, 1984

Pynoos R, Eth S: Witness to violence: the child interview. J Am Acad Child Psychiatry (in press)

Pynoos R, Gilmore K, Shapiro T: Children's response to parental suicide behavior. Presented at the annual meeting of the American Academy of Child Psychiatry, Dallas, 1981

Russell D: Rape in Marriage. New York, Macmillan, 1982

Shaffer D, Fisher P: The epidemiology of suicide in children and young adolescents. J Am Acad Child Psychiatry 20:545–565, 1981

Schetky PH: Preschoolers' responses to murder of their mothers by their fathers: a study of four cases. Bull Am Acad Psychiatry Law 6:45–57, 1973

Silverman D: Sharing the crisis of rape: counseling the mates and family members of victims. Am J Orthopsychiatry 1:166–173, 1978

Strauss M, Gelles R, Steinmetz S: Behind Closed Doors: Violence in the American Family. New York, Anchor Books, 1980

Terr L: Children of Chowchilla: study of psychic trauma. Psychoanal Study Child 34:547–623, 1979

Terr L: Chowchilla revisited: the effects of psychic trauma four years after a school bus kidnapping. Am J Psychiatry 140:1543–1550, 1983

Weissman M: The epidemiology of suicide attempts. Arch Gen Psychiatry 30:737–746, 1974

Wells A: No more victims: Carolyn Craven talks about rape, and about what women and men can do to stop it. Self-Determination Quarterly Journal 2:2, 1978

West LJ: The epidemic of violence. Presented at the annual meeting of the American Psychiatric Association, Los Angeles, May 1984

Chapter 3

Children Traumatized in Small Groups

Lenore Cagen Terr, M.D.

Chapter 3

Children Traumatized in Small Groups

S mall groups of youngsters who experience sudden, unexpected, intensely overwhelming external events either together or in tandem offer important opportunities for clinical study. By comparing individual children within such groups or among the different groups, investigators may learn about how a child's constitutional makeup, developmental stage, family, and past history influence the post-traumatic clinical picture. Psychiatrists may also discover which responses to psychic trauma occur regardless of the differences among individuals or groups. Studying small groups allows us to compare primary victims with witnesses and to differentiate the effects of single-blow trauma from those symptoms that result from repeated, chronic fright. We may eventually be able to compare the effects of sexual traumas with nonsexual ones. Most important, the underlying mechanisms of post-traumatic symptom formation may become more clear as we study and compare individuals within small groups of children who have experienced identical traumatic events.

This chapter reports a preliminary clinical investigation of four small groups of traumatized children, 15 youngsters ranging in age from 6 months to 12 years. Before I present these four groups, however, I will first deal with group phenomena and with the post-traumatic effects special to children, as opposed to adults, which I found in my field studies of 25 kidnapped youngsters from Chowchilla, California. I will then describe the four traumatic small-group situations, which are the focus of this chapter, and the youngsters who were involved in them. I will discuss the role of the group experience both as protective and as increasing vulnerabilities to post-traumatic symptoms. I will finally present five particularly striking new findings concerning the experience of certain children within these groups: 1) perception of ghosts; 2) misperception of time passage; 3) symbolization of the trauma in terms of the child's developmental phase, past experience, and inner life; 4) condensation

47

of trauma-related and other nonrelated ideas; and 5) formation of nonverbal memories. Because this chapter largely has to do with new data on childhood thinking and perception under severe stress, which was gathered by comparing the individual youngsters who sustained identical traumas within small groups, it will not even begin to cover many of the other questions regarding the group behaviors of traumatized clusters of children. Future research studies—including one currently in progress by the author of this chapter—may address some of these questions.

GROUPS AND THE CHOWCHILLA KIDNAPPING

In the late 1970s and early 1980s I studied the effects of a traumatic event—the kidnapping of an entire school bus of summer school students—upon the child victims, many of whom had not previously known each other well (Terr 1979). Throughout the 27-hour ordeal, the abductors treated the Chowchilla kidnap victims as a group. When I evaluated the kidnapped youngsters individually several months later, however, I found that while certain symptom categories (e.g., play, omens, foreshortened future, etc.) could be identified in most of the children, the special forms that these symptoms took were quite particular and specific to each individual child's personal past, family makeup, and developmental phase.

Symptom Contagion Within the Chowchilla Group

Certain post-traumatic symptoms seemed to spread quickly from child to child, affecting untraumatized siblings and family members and then the community-at-large; however, the same type of post-traumatic symptoms eventually came to affect two children who were entirely separated from their kidnapped peers quite soon after the event. Seven-year-old Sandra and eight-year-old Billy left Chowchilla, respectively, three months and one day after the traumatic event, and thus, they were relatively immune to symptoms spread by post-traumatic group interactions. Yet, entirely on their own, both Sandra and Billy developed omens, fourth-kidnapper fears (beliefs that someone in addition to the three jailed kidnappers had participated in the kidnapping and represented a present danger), post-traumatic play, and misperceptions or memories of misperceptions—the most contagious types of post-traumatic symptoms. Highly contagious symptoms were, therefore, also symptoms that easily could develop entirely independently in an individual child.

Group communications during the ordeal itself may have accounted for some of the symptoms that were widespread much later. A few post-traumatic ideas at Chowchilla probably *did* begin this way. For instance, three children spoke together about whether they would be shot one by one coming out of their van, and these three older Chowchilla victims later clung tenaciously to this frightening mental imagery. Three relatives—two sisters and a cousin—mentioned to one another either during the kidnapping or immediately afterwards arguments with their mothers that they had had, and these girls later all held strongly to their mutually communicated "omens."

On the other hand, some early or immediate potentially pathogenic communications were rejected by the group. It appeared that a symptom that was communicated within the Chowchilla group from one child to another would not take root unless it fell upon already receptive soil. Then, too, in and of themselves, some seeds lacked growing-power. Susan, five, described to her best friend Ellen, six, a visual hallucination of the kidnappers she had experienced while buried alive, but that particular symptom did not grow at all within the group. The hallucination was too elaborate, too extreme, and far too personally derived to be transplanted to the minds of the other youngsters. On the other hand, some such seed would sprout in almost any soil. Omens, for instance, reflected the almost universal readiness among the children to latch onto a "reason" that the whole thing happened, or a "turning point" which could have been avoided (18 children eventually "discovered" omens). Post-traumatic play, fears of extra kidnappers, and misperceptions were also easily transmitted from one child to another.

Lack of Group Cohesiveness at Chowchilla

Groups of traumatized Chowchilla youngsters avoided remaining in touch with one another after the event. For instance, Johnny and Debbie, who had been 5th-grade boyfriend–girlfriend before the kidnapping, "broke up" soon afterwards. Six-year-old Benji and his self-appointed object of concern during the kidnapping, Susan, five, did not maintain their relationship afterwards, even though Susan later told me that she felt quite grateful to Benji for his gallantry during their ordeal. (Benji had warned a kidnapper, "You better not touch Susan.") As a matter of fact, only two kidnapped schoolgirls remained close friends four to five years after the kidnapping, Ellen and Susan (six and five years old when they were kidnapped). This friendship flourished, despite Susan's grandmother's strongly stated objection—"Being friends when you are both kidnapped is wrong." Only one kidnapping reunion was ever held in Chowchilla—and this had been suggested and sponsored by an out-of-town group of benefactors.

This fragmentation of groupings, something Kai Erikson noted at Buffalo Creek (Erikson 1976), extended to the child victim's parents. An early attempt of some Chowchilla parents to set up an organization failed miserably. My own research and therapeutic Saturday morning parents' group meetings of 1977 were attended by the same five or six mothers, despite an invitation that had been extended by me to each one of the 14 families then residing in Chowchilla. When I returned in 1978 to read to the parents a first draft of my findings, only three of them came to hear it—and one of these mothers dropped by mainly to ask me about a new aspect of her son's behavior. One could not escape the observation that this group was assiduously avoiding "groupiness." Embarrassed and frightened about their own vulnerability and loss of control in the past, no one wished to be reminded of it. It is important to note that the Chowchilla victims and their families were able to assimilate into the normal community after their ordeal. Some victims of more chronic and dehumanizing experiences, such as the holocaust or the famines and wars of Southeast Asia cannot join into nonvictim society as well as the Chowchilla group did.

How was the group-avoidance at Chowchilla different from the behaviors of the many war veterans, who seem (at least in radio and TV reports) to thrive on combat-unit reunions and ceremonial visits to the old battlefields? I believe that the difference comes about because of a soldier's identity as a soldier and because of military training. Soldiers are exercised together, marched together, taught together, left alone at leisure together, and punished together enough to achieve significant group cohesiveness. They also establish an identity—both professional and personal—as military men. Military training forces enough education, physical fitness, quick reflexive behaviors, and endurance into oneself to prepare—at least in part—to mentally and physically survive the horrors of battle. Most soldiers will automatically behave during combat the way they were originally trained in camp to act. The vast majority of soldiers so trained will not become overwhelmingly stressed in war despite the occurrence of terrifying events. (Although they may harbor for years one or two symptoms related to combat—such as William Manchester's [1979] 30-year-old post-traumatic dream.) The fact that each soldier is expected to reintegrate quickly into ordinary postwar society after wartime ordeals probably helps the soldiers to overcome on their own or to "live with" some early or partial post-traumatic syndromes.

The most severe and totally unanticipated stresses *will* precipitate a fully developed post-traumatic stress disorder in the previously normal, well-trained, and reassimilated soldier. Unfortunately, there

are enough entirely unexpected and gruesomely dehumanizing occurrences during wartime to ensure that post-traumatic stress casualties will remain high, and as a matter of fact, keep coming to light
(Yager et al. 1984) long after the truces have been signed and the
diplomats have gone home.

Armed-forces training, in general, can mold a group cohesiveness
that lasts despite the impingement of highly stressful events upon
members of the group. In most peacetime disasters, however, with
no possibility of anticipating when and where the event will fall,
there is no way to prepare for the peril. These previously untrained
groups do not seek out reunions or develop cohesions. As a matter
of fact, they will avoid each other as symbols of their frightening
experience. Most humans will not voluntarily seek out reminders of
their exquisite vulnerabilities.

POST-TRAUMATIC STRESS DISORDER OF CHILDHOOD: FINDINGS FROM THE CHOWCHILLA GROUP—AGES 5–14

The Chowchilla field studies allowed the delineation of some manifestations of post-traumatic stress disorder that particularly mark the
response of children, as opposed to adults. These findings have been
confirmed in an increasing number of separately and individually
traumatized children whom I have been evaluating in my clinical
practice (now more than 50).

Children differ from adults following intense, unanticipated stresses
in that:

1. Those over age 3 or 4 do not become partly or fully amnesic
   regarding overwhelming external events. They do not employ
   the denial of external reality or the massive repression that has
   been reported in some adults (Horowitz 1976). Children under
   3 or 4 *do*, at times, tend to forget their traumas—some may
   do so because of the massive repressions normal in the first
   years of life—and some because the trauma occurred at a time
   when no adequate words or symbols to represent and record
   it had yet been acquired. I will cover part of this seemingly
   forgotten world of the preschool trauma victim in the section
   of this chapter entitled "Preverbal Memories." It is important
   to bear in mind, however, that some toddlers will remember,
   years afterwards, detail for detail, every aspect of a traumatic
   event. Gislason and Call (1982) demonstrated this in their
   report on 36-months-old and younger dog-bite victims, and I
   have seen similar particularly detailed remembrances 12 years

after a horrible accident, by a 15-year-old girl, who at 2½ suffered a crushed leg when a fork lift truck fell on her.

2. Children, as opposed to adults, do not demonstrate psychic numbing. Adults who exhibit numbing probably do so, in part, because of their denial of external reality and also, in part, as a response to the experience of dehumanizing and/or repeated disaster. Reports on concentration-camp victims (Krystal and Niederland 1968) and on the victims of Hiroshima (Lifton 1967) particularly emphasize this finding. Some authors reporting upon the personalities of battered children have noted emptiness of relationships (Yates 1981) or a frozen paralytic quality (Green 1983), which may be somewhat akin to the numbing of adults; however, child abuse is almost always chronic and repeated, somewhat expected by the child, and associated, as well, with ongoing parental neglect and/or pathological defensive displacement (Galdston 1965; Terr 1970; Green 1983). Further study of the differential effects of acute and chronic stresses in youngsters is urgently needed (Terr 1984a).

3. Children do not experience sudden, unexpected visual flashbacks that interrupt their behaviors or disrupt their concentration. Anna Freud and Dorothy Burlingham make the point that youngsters gradually develop the ability to fantasize (1942), and this may have something to do with some young children's lack of disturbance by flashback phenomena. Furthermore, latency-age children often daydream at will, so they can *consciously* choose to think of their old ordeals. Willed, conscious daydreaming may partly block the chances for gruesome visions suddenly to intrude. In other words, voluntarily bringing on a vision may somewhat overcome the tendency of "dammed-up" visions to burst in upon their host. Probably the best reason children do not experience flashbacks is that since youngsters do not deny the external realities of a trauma, they do not experience what Horowitz (1976) conceives of as an alternating pattern of intrusions and massive denial.

4. Children's work performance (school) rarely suffers for more than a few months after psychic trauma, as opposed to the long-term decline in work efforts experienced by many adults. This relative childhood immunity to work inhibition most likely directly relates to the lack of denial, intrusive flashbacks, and psychic numbing in youngsters.

The fifth through seventh differences between childhood and adult responses to psychic trauma are mainly differences of frequency and intensity of symptomatology. Some adults *do* exhibit these same changes, but they do so less often or less blatantly than children do. These three types of behaviors do not massively change adult personalities, but they frequently account for personality shifts in children.

5. Post-traumatic play and reenactment occur much more frequently in childhood. These bear heavily upon the later personality development of the traumatized child.
6. Time skew is more common and more dramatically expressed in youngsters (Terr 1983c).
7. A foreshortened view of the future is a particularly striking post-traumatic manifestation of childhood trauma, although this blunting of temporal perspective is also frequently observed in traumatized adults (Terr 1984b). Children may act upon these limited future views (see Terr 1983b for some discussion of the limited future expectations in a normal control group randomly selected and then matched to the children of Chowchilla).

THE SMALL GROUPS

Group 1

The four Harrison children, Holly, 4 years 11 months; Duane, 4 years 1 month; Cindy, 7; and Winifred, 2, were swimming at their local pool complex when Holly slid away a metal cover guarding the kiddie pool's suction apparatus, put some little stones inside, sat down, and had her intestines literally sucked down the drain. Her father rushed over from the adult pool, shouted for the lifeguard to shut the pump, and wrapped Holly's protruding lengths of gut into a towel. (He was quite certain that only Duane had seen what happened, but I later learned from Cindy that she, too, had seen it.)

Two years after the accident Holly died in Pittsburgh, within hours of receiving a liver and intestinal transplant. Holly had been my psychiatric patient for the year before she died, and Cindy, Duane, and Winifred worked with me therapeutically both before and after Holly died. Despite the fact that they had heard some warnings to this effect from me, the Harrison children had not really expected Holly, who had already bravely sustained her injuries for two years, to die. Nine months after Holly's death in Pennsylvania, the family moved to England.

Group 2

Three families placed their youngsters in a day care home under the care of Mrs. Mary Beth Hillgard. Unbeknownst to the families, Leroy Hillgard, Mary Beth's husband, used these youngsters for pornographic photographs—some alone, and some in lewd acts or poses with each other or with him. Almost three years after the children had been under Mrs. Hillgard's care, Leroy was arrested by customs agents who had been watching for him for some time. The parents, who had not known at all up to this time that their children had been sexually misused, learned about it from the police. Three of the children were definitely identified by their parents from their pornographic pictures (Gloria Rivers, who was 0–6-months-old when she stayed at the Hillgards' home, and her half brother, Joe Hillgard, 0–36-months-old during the time the Hillgards cared for him, both Mr. Hillgard's stepgrandchildren; and Sarah Fellows, 15–18-months-old while she was a day care attendee). The other three youngsters showed, on psychiatric examination, that they, too, had been exposed in some way to Mr. Hillgard's sexual attention (Brent Burns, 3–24-months-old at the Hillgards' nursery; Morton Fellows, 3 years 6 months to 3 years 9 months, at the Hillgards' home; and Paul Fellows, 5 years 7 months to 5 years 10 months, while under the Hillgards' care).

The frightening situation in the Hillgards' Day Care Center was most likely a series of events, rather than one single, shocking, and unanticipated blow.

Group 3

Jonathan Burgess, 12, had been "grounded" by his mother for failing to finish his homework. He returned home immediately after school and within minutes an escaped murderer, Albert, on the run from an Alabama penal institution, pulled into the driveway in a stolen car. Albert rang the bell, put a knife to Jonathan's throat, tied the child up, and held him hostage. Soon afterwards, James, Jonathan's 9-year-old brother, and their friend Howard, 11½, came home, too. The convict applied identical treatment to these latecomers.

The three boys were held 11 hours, while Albert negotiated with the police. Jonathan suddenly worked up an escape scheme, driven into action by an attempt on Albert's part to fondle his genitals. The Burgess boys and their friend bolted from the house and ran to safety. Albert was almost immediately arrested. Jonathan was acknowledged by all to be a hero. I interviewed the brothers, Jonathan and James, twice—first six weeks after the event and again, 19 months afterwards.

Group 4

The three Lee boys, Peter, 12, Manuel, 10, and Isaac, 8, were doing Peter's paper route one afternoon in a quiet California central valley town when Isaac asked his older brothers if he could toss the news-papers at a few houses on the route directly across Logan Avenue. Returning to join his siblings, Isaac carefully looked before crossing the wide street but was suddenly struck by a speeding car, seemingly coming from nowhere. He was rendered totally paralyzed from his neck down. Manuel saw the entire incident, but Peter had turned his head away for an instant, so that he saw only Isaac's body being dragged and the horrible aftermath.

Isaac was in a coma for a week and he remained in hospitals for the next nine months. When he returned home he required nurses around-the-clock and continued breathing assistance through a trach-eostomy tube. He was able to talk, with some difficulty, and he could write, steer his wheelchair, and draw, using solely his mouth and his chin muscles. Because of the initial severe swelling of his brain and the shock and the concussion, Isaac could remember nothing what-soever of his afternoon on the Logan Avenue paper route.

(*Note*: The Harrison, Burgess, Fellows, Burns, Hillgard, Rivers, and Lee children are part of an expanding group of single cases and identical traumatized groups I have evaluated and/or treated in my psychiatric practice. The children's names are uniformly disguised, so that they may be recognized in any other publications in which they appear. Recently I have added fictitious last names, in order to aid the reader in keeping so many children straight. If the reader is interested in Holly Harrison for instance, he or she will find mention of Holly in articles written prior to mid-1984 and Holly Harrison or Holly H. in papers written thereafter. The same children appear in more than one publication because some of them exemplify more than one new finding having to do with such phenomena as post-traumatic play, time distortion, and/or post-traumatic cognition and memory.)

GROUP PHENOMENA IN THE FOUR SMALL GROUPS

Failure of Child Victims and Child Witnesses to Communicate Verbally

In each of these four traumatic episodes, sets of siblings experienced the events together, yet they did not admit recall, or reveal to me that they talked much with one another about their shared experi-ences. Isaac Lee said that he asked his brother Manuel *once* what had happened to him, and he had told him. But Isaac went on to say that they had not discussed the accident ever again. Manuel and Peter did not discuss the incident together either.

The two Hillgard grandchildren, who had been sexual victims at day care, were not observed by their mother discussing, playing out, or reenacting their sexual experiences together, even though their mother saw Joe exposing neighborhood children to his overtly excited gestures, dance, and masturbation. The Fellows youngsters, who also had been victims of Mr. Hillgard, did not appear to have talked about their ordeals with one another. The two Fellows brothers both became unusually modest after their stay at the day care facility, but this trait was far more prominent in the older boy. Paul most likely began employing this type of defensive behavior first, and then Morton imitated him. Mr. and Mrs. Fellows did not see or hear their children discussing anything about the Hillgards, with the exception of some frequently offered complaints about Mary Beth's cooking. Leroy's name never seemed to come up among the children.

The Burgess boys had experienced an adventure—scary though it was—and they were celebrated throughout their neighborhood. Despite the appealing cops-and-robbers aspects to their story, however, they did not talk much together about their shared experience. Their small group, like the others, was a relatively silent one. The Burgesses *did* find one hostage-related activity they liked to share: listening to Albert's voice on tape. But the two boys listened so much that Mr. Burgess "lost" the tape, on purpose. The tapes had not served, however, as a stimulus for the boys to converse among themselves. Jonathan did not tell his brother about Albert's sexual advances, and James did not relate to his sibling an omen he had constructed, in which each year would start out with a fresh disaster.

Of course the above observations are informal, and the youngsters might, indeed, have talked together secretly. Yet the siblings whom I knew best because I followed the youngsters in treatment for well over a year—the Harrison children—similarly did not verbally share their pain with one another. Before Holly's death, the family had taken a stoic nonverbal approach to the horrors of Holly's accident and the illness, because they wanted Holly to remain in good spirits, and they felt that they could not risk even the smallest amount of flagging in her will to live. They *believed* she would live. After Holly's death, the young Harrisons continued their relatively nonverbal course despite their mother's willingness and interest in talking with them. Duane, particularly close to Holly, could not share his feelings with his other siblings. When Winifred talked, she confided only to her mother—not to the other affected siblings. When Cindy talked—

only once in the first half-year after Holly's death—she exposed her feelings to a grandmother visiting from across the sea. Duane barely talked about his pain, yet he was the most profoundly affected child in the family.

These sibling groups could not be compared with nonsibling small groups who were traumatized, because no small groups of separate youngsters came to me for evaluation and study. But the reader may recall the Chowchilla group was composed of both sibling groups and individuals, and most of these did not like to discuss their reactions to the kidnapping whether or not they were with siblings at the time of the frightening event.

Relative Noncontagion of Post-Traumatic Symptoms Within the Small Groups

Post-traumatic play (Terr 1981), reenactment, fears, and omen formation symptoms were as common among these 15 children as they were at Chowchilla. Yet it was interesting to note that affected siblings preferred to play post-traumatically with outsiders rather than with their co-victim siblings. Manuel Lee, for example, repeatedly played Car-crash and Ambulance with his friend Jeremiah, but he played only standard football games with his older brother and co-witness Peter. When Jonathan Burgess went out for the first time to dodge cars and "tee pee" (toilet paper) houses—a post traumatic game for him because he had wished to dodge the convict Albert's car—he did not include his younger brother and co-victim, James. It was only later, when this post-traumatic dodging and tee-peeing routine had infected the entire neighborhood, that James was also included. The Fellows and the Hillgard children, both highly affected by their sexual abuse at the day care program, never played sexual games together. Even though the older Hillgard boy exposed his neighborhood peers to highly sexualized dances, he did not show these to his little sister. His post-traumatic games were played secretly with nontraumatized peers. Two of the Fellows siblings drew nude, sexual pictures of adults at school, but the youngsters had studied in separate classrooms, and their mother never found any mutually designed drawings at home.

I was able to treat each of the Harrison children, and this more-extensive observational opportunity confirmed my impression that traumatized siblings do not ordinarily share together in post-traumatic play. (One exception to this tendency was found at Chowchilla. Elizabeth and Mary played Kidnap Tag together for four to five years, although each girl also played a secret, separate, and entirely individual game during the same period.) Cindy, the oldest child witness to Holly Harrison's evisceration, habitually wound up strings and ropes, or she tied these intestine-like materials onto bedposts and doorknobs, making a massive gut web of her room. Duane, on the other hand, repeatedly built round swimming pools and little drains with his blocks. Holly, too, played when she felt up to it. She ate small stones (what she had been putting into the drain before it sucked her in), and she buried tiny rocks in holes all around the house and yard. Here, then, were three affected siblings, each playing a separately invented, post-traumatic game. No mutual sharing seemed to take place—with one interesting exception. All four Harrisons including Winifred, the spared toddler, played Hospital together. In my opinion, this was not post-traumatic play, it was more ordinary child's play geared to work through the continually changing, chronic stresses of Holly's longstanding illness and her hospitalizations. The children's Hospital plots frequently changed, reflecting the changing picture of Holly's medical treatments. When Holly died, Hospital stopped. The Harrison children had been able to share in ordinary child's play, but they could not show each other their very secretive inner worlds, their post-traumatic play. Cindy's separate game of string-winding lasted months after Holly's death, despite numerous psychotherapeutic interpretations with which Cindy, at least vocally, agreed.

In the case of the other, less-observable or less-striking post-traumatic changes, it was harder to discern how shared attitudes within small groupings influenced the individual child. There was no sibling-to-sibling transmission of James Burgess's omen connecting seasonal beginnings and disaster, nor was there any spread of Manuel Lee's conviction that he would live only to age 40 to his brother, Peter, who told me he'd live to age 70. But, on the other hand, Isaac Lee, who had been rendered totally paralyzed, told me that he could not at all envision growing up to adulthood. Had he conveyed some of this doomed feeling to Manuel? I could not tell. Such future foreshortening can crop up entirely unaided (Terr 1983a), so that group influences could not be dissected away from individual propensities. Each of the Lee boys felt afraid of strangers, but again, one could not determine whether group or individual factors explained why each boy held the fear. A stranger in a car had hit Isaac. Why not develop a fear of strangers entirely unaided by group processes? This is the problem in understanding how group process influences the individual child victims within that group. One cannot clearly discern between the group and the separate individual determinants.

PROTECTION OR INCREASED VULNERABILITY FROM GROUP EXPERIENCE

These four small groups do not provide a definitive answer to how groups protect, make more vulnerable the traumatized individuals within them, or both. There was no help or hindrance afforded after a trauma by socializing with other victims because nonrelatives in the traumatized small groups did not continue their associations with one another. The Hillgard sex-victims did not continue playing together, although Brent Burns, Morton Fellows, and Joe Hillgard separately mentioned in their interviews the Star Wars Games that they had played at day care (probably a Leroy Hillgard-inspired sex-variation on the George Lucas theme), as well as some remembrances of their playmates—the other two boys. Perhaps each little boy found some relief from early post-traumatic guilt by realizing that other boys, whom they still remembered, also played the same "games" that they had played with Leroy. Groups of nonrelated adults, whom I examined after an airplane crash and a freak swimming pool electrocution, did not keep in touch with one another afterwards. They seemed to find no support from the others in their traumatized group, but rather reported experiencing relief at having family members or old friends arrive at the scene. Once overwhelmed, an individual has very little capacity to help others who are also being psychologically overcome. A person may find some solace in seeing that everyone else "in the same boat" is emotionally paralyzed or ineffective, but panic easily breeds under the identical circumstances.

Grinker and Spiegel's World War II studies of *traumatic neuroses* in soldiers (1945) showed that the best treatment at that time consisted of quick evacuation away from the front, brief abreactive treatment, and early integration back into the nontraumatized general unit. Trauma victims may unknowingly replicate this plan of action by automatically seeking reintegration into their families and neighborhoods, avoiding most contacts with their fellows-in-trauma. This may be helpful, although the data are not in.

Since each traumatic situation is different, a clarification of group-protectiveness from, versus group-enhancement of, vulnerability in trauma awaits a careful study investigating similar events experienced both by separate individuals and by small groups. Even with such a research design, however, the answer may be difficult to obtain.

GHOSTS

After traumatic events that lead to the death of a close friend or a family member, the survivor victims or survivor witnesses may "see" or "feel" their dead associate.

Although the idea of post-traumatic ghosts may sound quite familiar to the theatergoer (Shakespeare's *Hamlet* and *Macbeth*, for instance) or to the opera fan (Mozart's *Don Giovanni*), *ghosts* or *presences* have not been fully explored by psychologists and psychiatrists. Ghosts frequently occur in the anthropological literature—for instance, in Freeman et al.'s (1976) studies of Apaches—and also in the literature of early normal child development (Shapiro et al. 1980); but they have not, from my readings of the psychic-trauma literature, been connected before to psychic trauma. Parkes, in a study of London widows within the first year of their husbands' deaths, noted that some widows sensed their husbands' presences. On the other hand, Parkes did not connect this phenomenon to trauma nor did he differentiate which of the husbands had died unexpectedly or shockingly. Parkes reached the conclusion that only a few of the more psychologically disturbed widows sensed their husbands' presences (Parkes 1970).

The Harrison children who experienced their eviscerated sister's presence were four and seven years old at the time they did so. Although I have not heard of ghosts visiting any child younger than four, several adults have reported this phenomenon to me after the shocking death of a person who had been important to them. Neither Duane, seven, nor Winifred, four, referred to Holly's sensed presence as a ghost, but their descriptions are the stuff of which ghost stories are made. These kinds of post-traumatic misperceptions may eventually account for the phenomenon of ghost sightings, which is so much a part of our cultural and social heritage. In reading my quotes from Duane and Winifred Harrison, the moviegoer may be reminded of the 10-year-old Alexander of Bergman's *Fanny and Alexander*, whose father dies suddenly and traumatically and whose subsequent days and months are marked by repeated, vivid sightings of his father's ghost.

First, let us hear from Winifred at age four—two months after Holly died. "My sister lives in a children's cemetery and she plays every day with the other children buried there. . . . She comes to me in my sleep *and* with my eyes open. . . . She wants to play with me. I'm frightened. I don't want to play. . . ." A few months later Winifred told me, "Holly's the angel on my Christmas tree," and "Mousie [Holly's favorite toy from my office] is in a tree and only me, Grandma, and Grandpa can see her. The others cannot. I lost a balloon and Grandma told me that Holly would catch it above the clouds. . . . Mousie is watching everything." I worked therapeutically with Winifred, talking with her and playing, about her pre-sleep hallucinations of Holly, her dreams of Holly's invitations to play, and her sense (inspired by Grandma) that Holly was still watching her. By six months following Holly's death, Winifred seemed to have stopped "seeing" her dead sister. A letter Winifred's mother sent me from England nine months after Holly's death indicated that, indeed, Winnie no longer was bothered by visits from Holly.

Duane never thought that he could "see" Holly; he "felt" her instead. Seven months after Holly died, Duane told his mother that he was hoping the weather would be nice for a weekend family trip to Disneyland, but, "Holly plays tricks. It would be just like her to make it rain at Disneyland." He went on to elaborate. "She makes the doors close behind me when I don't want them closed." Duane and Holly had been born only 10 months apart and were more like twins than siblings. They shared a secret language and committed frequent pranks during Holly's short lifetime. The close relationship itself and the traumatic way that Holly was injured and had died led to Duane's sense that his sister was still with him. Grandma's comments may have further magnified this tendency.

Ghosts may turn out to be fairly common post-traumatic findings when trauma is connected with the shocking death of a loved one. In most ghost stories, the ghost wanders about because something is left unresolved after a sudden and premature death. Of course, this lack of resolution is really an internal problem of the ghost storyteller, not the ghost. Ghosts depend upon post-traumatic misperception and hallucination for their very existence. None of the small groups I evaluated that were involved in a psychic trauma unconnected to death saw ghosts afterwards. Furthermore, since Winifred's and Duane's ghostlike visitations were quite different in form and in content, they most likely did not spread through sibling influence. There was only one detail in both the Harrison children's ghost stories which, in each case, seemed to have spread from Grandma's openly stated belief—the idea that Holly was somewhere above them watching everyone.

TIME DISTORTION

The finding in these small groups that there were various problems with time sense confirms and furthers the observations that I have been making, starting with the Chowchilla studies. There are difficulties in perceiving and appreciating time during the following severe, unexpected stresses (Teer 1983b). Although we know that children's operations regarding time are not fully developed before age 12 (Piaget 1927), the time distortions that the children experiencing small-group traumas reported went well past simple immaturities.

During their 11-hour incarceration, Jonathan and James Burgess, the 9- and 11-year old hostages, partially lost their ability to be aware of natural internal rhythms in order to tell the time. (In nontraumatic circumstances, this type of time sense stays intact because individuals are able to perceive their own biorhythms [Halberg 1969]). Albert, the convict, had cut the electrical wires into the house, so that the clocks were not working. Jonathan told me after Albert's trial, "The public defender tried to make us seem like liars. He asked, "What time?' There were no clocks. I said, "4 o'clock.' He said, "How do you know?' He asked the same questions three or four times."

"He did the same to me," James added.

"I feel he might have been successful in that," Jonathan went on slowly and thoughtfully. "He tried to make me dumb."

Jonathan did indeed *feel* dumb and inept about time during the trial. It was not the public defender, but Jonathan's and James's overwhelming anxiety during their ordeal that led to their confusion about the times of day. The failure to perceive the correct time under traumatic circumstances should be seen as a confirmation that the witness has been traumatized rather than a way to discredit the young victim on the witness stand.

Turning back the clock—or at least the wish to do so—was another time-distortive phenomenon frequently observed in these traumatized youngsters. Duane Harrison, at five, and Cindy, at eight and a half, often thought about the old days in New York before Holly was injured. Their mother said, "Cindy sits down and cries and says, 'I miss Joanna so much.' It's like she's trying to turn back time. . . . Duane, too, says he wishes to return to New York. Holly, also, talks about her best friend in New York, who was not a close friend at all. . . . It's like a collective kind of thought."

Duane told me, "Sometimes I wish to go back to New York. If we went back, Holly wouldn't be sick. She would have to be better when we go out there. She won't be sick. Otherwise we can't go there."

In her own session, Cindy Harrison, well into latency, sounded less primitive than her brother, but still quite magical in her wishes to turn back time. "I think things wouldn't have happened," she said, "if we had stayed in New York. I kind of think of New York as a place where bad things don't happen."

Not only did the clock turn back for the traumatized youngsters, but it could turn forward. Little Brent Burns, who between 3 and 24 months of age was the victim of adult sexual assaults, was totally confused about forward- and backward-moving time at age 4. He told me, the first time that we met, "I used to be 17. I turned back to 4. My heart went clanggg. That's all I can say." Not only was young Brent confused about the direction of time progression, but his former and current behaviors had become designated by the ages that he felt were appropriate for certain sexual activities. Brent felt he had been "older" sexually as a toddler than he was now as a preschooler—and his apparent confusion was unconsciously expressing this self-perception.

One last and, unfortunately, frequently observed difficulty in this group was a foreshortening of the future or a sense of lack of future possibilities. For instance, Sarah Fellows, sexually abused between 15 and 18 months of age by Leroy Hillgard, said about her own future, at age 5: "I'll live probably to 40 or 49. When you're old you'll die....My grandparents—they're older than 49 and I don't think *they're* ready to die. Sometimes I think I'm going to die sooner than other people. I don't know why I think this. I want to be a nurse. I'm *never* going to be in the army. I feel the future is dangerous. You could die. I feel bad people will hurt me. I may be killed instead of dying. You don't come back after you die. In armies they have guns and can shot—shoot people. I kind of feel there was danger at Mary Beth Hillgard's house, but I don't know what it was."

SYMBOLIZATION AND CONDENSATION

Although trauma can be defined as an experience that is taken in intact and leaves an indigestible mental image (this conception comes from Robert Michels, M.D., New York), some parts of the trauma may eventually be symbolically reprocessed. Portions of the traumatic imagery may also become amalgamated, or condensed, with other nontraumatic mental representations. Through interpreting symbols and condensations we can observe how phase-specific, developmental features are added to a child's memories and impressions of traumatic events, one way in which traumatic impressions are individually unique even though they were once experienced within a group.

Five-year-old Holly Harrison, who later died, exemplifies how symbolization and condensation of traumatic images occur. I saw this effect in Holly as I treated her whenever she felt well enough to come to my office the year before she died, and I learned a great deal about the inner workings of little Holly's mind. She was preoccupied with oedipal issues at 4 years 11 months when she was eviscerated. For this small girl, the injuring drain represented a male. The tubes the doctors inserted, likewise, became male symbols—snakes. She described her evisceration a year after the accident, "I was sitting there like a table and I was trying to get off, but *he* was pulling me so hard." Holly's drain was a "he."

Mr. Harrison recalled, on a different occasion, that "she really hated the tubes in her tummy after the operation. She said, 'I don't want a snake in my tummy which keeps biting me.' It was *her* idea, that snake. The tube was put in under general anesthesia. She hated it there. She had never been really afraid of snakes, but she had said 'yukky' at a snake once."

Holly mentioned a "witch" to me directly after she spoke of the "male" drain in the swimming pool. "There have been more things more frightening," she said. "At night when I lie there, a witch would come by my window and push it through. I think that every night. She'd steal my toys. She would take my tubes [Holly's snake] away and put it in her broom. I had this [the witch idea] *before* the accident."

Her mother, who was sitting in, interrupted. "She *never* talked about it before." Holly apparently had skewed time, misplacing thoughts that had come afterward into a preceding position.

"Later, in the hospital," Holly went on, "I thought of witches. My daydream made it up. But *now* I think it [the fantasy] happened before, and the witch made it [the accident] happen."

Holly's witch and snake were five-year-old symbolic impressions of her parents. The witch would lurk near Holly's bed hoping to steal Holly's snake—now her lifeline intravenous tubes—away from her. In Holly's mind, this vengeful female could loose untold pain and misery upon her. The snake—though originally feared, for his biting and pulling—was now loved and urgently necessary to Holly. Holly's trauma had quickly taken on an oedipal flavor through her incorporation of oedipal phase-specific symbols into the traumatic imagery. Her condensation of drains, abdominal tubes, and parenteral feeding tubes into one male symbol—the snake—had abbreviated a number of concerns, both real and imaginary, into one single image.

Not only developmental phase but the child's past history could color mental representations of a traumatic occurrence. James, nine years old when he was kidnapped, hadn't begun speaking until well after age three. He had needed a few years of speech therapy as a preschooler for a muscle-related problem. In first grade, James was found not to auditorially discriminate between sounds well, and he received considerable special tutoring in reading as a result. When Albert kidnapped him, this much-tutored boy did some immediate thinking. "I never thought I'd die," he told me. "I thought he'd brainwash me like Patty Hearst." The brainwashing idea had stemmed from all the speech and language help that James had endured. In his own view, James indeed *had* been brainwashed.

Condensations are not always easy to detect in waking mental life.

Thus I found the following exchange with four-year-old Winifred Harrison quite interesting. Young Winnie, who at two had been spared the sight of Holly's evisceration, at four had had to go through enormous shock and grief when Holly suddenly died as the doctors attempted a massive transplantation procedure in Pennsylvania. About six months after Holly's death, the Harrisons decided to move to England, and Winifred knew all about it. I thought we had better talk about the family move, but Winnie anticipated me. She bounded into my office and immediately began loading up all my trucks with tiny dolls.

"They're going to Pittsburgh," the sprite-like child piped.

"Where Holly died?" I asked.

"Yes. But they are going to a show. Nobody dies," she assured me. Winnie then carefully separated Holly's favorite toy, Mousie, from the group of dolls on trucks, who were moving away. "Mousie will be left here." she announced. "He will take care of hisself. The family is moving," she directly went on to explain, like a little schoolteacher. "To Pittsburgh. Pittsburgh. They are moving in April."

Winifred had in one deft mental stroke combined Holly's death site and, perhaps, the heaven that death site may have symbolized to Winnie, with the place at the opposite side of the globe to which her family would really be moving. The two ideas, quite removed, were being brought together into one symbol—a thought condensation—*Pittsburgh*.

It is my impression that mental condensations are more obvious and plentiful in the waking thoughts of children below ages four or five than they are in the waking states of older children and adults, but they are certainly evident in the dreams of both adults and children.

PREVERBAL MEMORIES

Probably the most fascinating single finding from these small groups was the type of memory still evident in children who were traumatized prior to the establishment of any real verbal ability. The three youngest children at the Hillgards' Day Care Center—Gloria (0–6 months), Sarah (15–18 months), and Brent (3–24 months) each could produce no recollections in my office in response to such questions as "Did you ever go to somebody's house for babysitting?" or "Do you remember the Hillgards?" or "Tell me about your babysitters." Yet they demonstrated for me a striking kind of perceptual memory of the trauma, through their play in the office or through the fears that they described. Two-year-old Gloria smothered my small dolls with much heavier dolls, with blankets, or with cars and trucks that she placed over them (like adults on top of children). She jabbed her finger into the "vagina" of a doll immediately upon undressing it. She poked this doll, as she looked about my room, seemingly trying to determine when I would be looking away.

Brent, at four, constructed a hotel in my office where, he said, "Movies are being made." He set up a line of truck drivers waiting to get into the hotel. "They take pictures with their clothes off," he explained as he played. "They like to. . . . The children fight and play around. The parents also have their clothes off. They sometimes make their picture, too, without clothes. . . . They are Gumdrop Grandma and Gumdrop Grandpa. . . . The children like taking the pictures. They get excited. Then their penis unties—looses off. It comes off their bodies. They like to lose their penis. Then they get it back. The people at the hotel run and run to get it [the lost penis]. . . . When the children stop playing, fussing, and taking pictures, their penis gets very softer. When do I get out of here? . . . The guy in the car carrier is late. He's naked. The hotel is closed. The truck drivers are going to fight and fuss. They're going to play with *his* penis. The Grandma wouldn't, but the Grandpa *would*. The guy in the car carrier likes it. Grandpa Gumdrop plays with his penis. . . . The guy is real quiet on the truck now that he has played. He's stopped talking." (In actuality, Brent's speech, which had developed early, entirely ceased for several months when he turned two.)

In four psychiatric sessions with me and in one with another child psychiatrist, Brent Burns demonstrated absolutely no verbal memory of the ordeal, which he must have experienced between 3 and 24 months of age. He could not remember the Hillgards at all. He listed babysitters who watched him from age 3 on, in response to any questions about sitters or day care. Yet Brent's play almost exactly duplicated much of what had probably happened to him. Brent's still-operational 2-year-old interpretations of adult sexuality: "fighting, fussing, and playing"; and his castration fears: "their penis looses off"; were firmly affixed to the prekindergartner's original perceptions of the trauma. Brent's play seemed to me like a slightly disguised post-traumatic dream. A few symbolic elaborations had adhered to the traumatic imagery, but Brent's mental representation of his days at the Hillgard day care nursery appeared barely altered from what would have been waking post-traumatic memories in an older child. Brent's memories were entirely unconscious.

Sarah Fellows, at five, could not remember the Hillgards either. But Sarah's nonretrievable memories took the form of fears instead of post-traumatic play. In my office the kindergartner told me,

I'm afraid of some things but I don't know what they are. I used to be scared of a cow. I never saw one. Moo-oo-oo-oo! I thought that part [she hand-motioned the udder] was really scary too. It looked like some kind of monster to me when I was little. I also remember we went on a boat in Disneyland—an animal boat—some have stripes. We saw lots of animals. Some little Indians popped up with spears. and I was scared of *that*."

Somebody scared me once with a finger part. I *can't* remember. *I'm afraid of a finger part on my stomach.* Right here. [She pointed at her upper abdomen, and fixed me with her gaze. *This* was important to Sarah.]

I'm afraid of sharp fingernails. I like ladies better than men—women better than men. Boys are really strong. I like girls who are not really strong too much.

I surmised that this child had feared penises (a finger-part) for many years as a result of her experiences with Leroy Hillgard, and I guessed that she had also displaced the origional area of assault upwards from her genitals to her abdomen. Sarah's father showed me, however, that the second part of my hypothesis was wrong.

I asked Sarah's father after Sarah's session exactly what the pornographic photograph the police had shown him of Sarah had depicted. "Hillgard's penis was touching the upper part of Sarah's abdomen," he said. "And Sarah was crying."

Sarah had pointed to her body when she told me "I'm afraid of a finger part on my stomach." The place she had pointed to had been the upper part of her abdomen—the very same anatomical area that Leroy Hillgard had assaulted and had photographed.

These quite precise nonverbal memories impressed me with how early in life traumatic impressions can be laid down, how close to the actual traumatic event these perceptual "memories" remain, and how vulnerable to trauma a child with little-to-no cognitive understanding of life events can be. Perception is more basic and primitive than is cognition. Once a traumatic perception is taken in, it may forever remain an "indigestible" part of the growing young personality.

SUMMARY

I have presented data regarding the experiences of children traumatized within groups. In addition I have contributed a preliminary report of five types of post-traumatic thinking evident in the 15 children studied, following their being in small groups which were severely stressed. Some youngsters who were exposed to overwhelming events connected with deaths experienced perceptual distortions akin to ghost sightings. Several others experienced disturbances of time sense. The disordered time perceptions included in this report went well beyond simple developmental immaturities. The traumatized youngsters in this series of cases, furthermore, tended to experience their trauma in terms of their developmental stages or past conflicts. Symbols of these were integrated with their mental representations of the trauma. Two youngsters who were studied over time were found to condense two entirely separate issues into one mental representation, which combined together because of associational similarities and/or wishes. Finally, the three youngest children in this series, who could not at all verbalize what had happened to them, demonstrated quite precise and long-lasting perceptual "memories" of the traumatic event, exhibited entirely through their play or through their fears. The traumatic origins of these phenomena remained entirely unconscious both to the youngsters and to their families.

Looking at small groups gives the psychiatric observer a meaningful opportunity to compare individuals who experience the same traumatic event. This opportunity makes it possible to delineate new findings and to clarify further the psychological effects of severe fright and externally generated stress.

REFERENCES

Erikson K: Everything in Its Path. New York, Simon and Schuster, 1976

Freeman D, Foulks E, Freeman P: Ghost sickness and superego development in the Kiowa Apache male, in The Psychoanalytic Study of Society, vol. 7. Edited by Muenstergerger W. Clinton, Mass, The Colonial Press, 1976

Freud A, Burlingame D (1942): Report 12, in the writings of Anna Freud, vol. 3. New York, International Universities Press, 1973

Galdston R: Observations of children who have been physically abused and their parents. Am J Psychiatry 122:440–443, 1965

Gislason L, Call J: Dog-bite in infancy: trauma and personality development. J Am Acad Child Psychiatry 21:203–207, 1982

Green A: Psychological trauma in abused children. J Am Acad Child Psychiatry 22:231–237, 1983

Grinker R, Spiegel J: Men under Stress. Philadelphia, Blakiston, 1945

Halberg, F: Chronobiology. Annual Review of Physiology 31:675–725, 1969

Horowitz M: Stress-Response Syndromes. New York, Jason Aronson, 1976

Krystal H, Niederland W: Clinical observations on the survivor syndrome, in Massive Psychic Trauma. Edited by Krystal H. New York, International Universities Press, 1968

Lifton R: Death in Life: Survivors of Hiroshima. New York, Random House, 1967

Manchester W: Goodbye Darkness. Boston, Little, Brown and Co., 1979

Parkes C: The first year of bereavement. Psychiatry 33:444–467, 1970

Piaget J: The Child's Conception of Time (1927). New York, Ballantine Books, 1971

Shapiro T, Sherman M, Osowsky I: Preschool children's conception of ghosts. J Am Acad Child Psychiatry 19:41–55, 1980

Terr L: A family study of child abuse. Am J Psychiatry 127:665–671, 1970

Terr L: Children of Chowchilla: a study of psychic trauma. Psychoanal Study Child 34:547–623, 1979

Terr L: "Forbidden games"; post-traumatic child's play. J Am Acad Child Psychiatry 20:741–760, 1981

Terr L: Chowchilla revisited: the effects of psychic trauma four years after a school-bus kidnapping. Am J Psychiatry 140:1543–1550, 1983a

Terr L: Life attitudes, dreams, and psychic trauma in a group of "normal" children. J Am Acad Child Psychiatry 22:221–230, 1983b

Terr L: Time sense following psychic trauma: a clinical study of 10 adults and 20 children. Am J Orthopsychiatry 53:244–261, 1983c

Terr L: Children at risk: psychic trauma, in Psychiatry Update, vol. 3. Edited by Grinspoon L. Washington, DC, American Psychiatric Association, 1984a

Terr L: Time and trauma. Psychoanal Study Child 39:633–665, 1984b

Yager T, Laufer R, Gallops M: Some problems associated with war experience in men of the Viet Nam generation. Arch Gen Psychiatry 41:327–333, 1984

Yates A: Narcissistic traits in certain abused children. Am J Orthopsychiatry 51:55–62, 1981

Chapter 4

Children Traumatized by Catastrophic Situations

Calvin J. Frederick, Ph.D.

Chapter 4

Children Traumatized by Catastrophic Situations

This chapter focuses essentially upon the development of post-traumatic stress disorder (PTSD) in a variety of traumatic and catastrophic situations, with particular emphasis upon problems occurring in children. The experiences discussed are based upon a wide spectrum of calamitous events including natural and human-induced disasters, hostage taking, child molestation, and physical assault. PTSD can develop on a group or an individual basis, affecting both adults and children. In our studies, the latter includes anyone under 18 years of age. The following areas constitute the thrust of this article: (*a*) background and literature review of natural disasters and other stressful events, (*b*) comparisons of stressors studied by the author, and (*c*) considerations for intervention.

BACKGROUND AND LITERATURE REVIEWS

The appearance of PTSD among children has recently come into sharper focus with the recognition that this is a real problem of importance for younger persons as well as adults. The formulation and introduction of the new diagnostic entity of post-traumatic stress disorder first appeared in 1980 in the third edition of the *Diagnostic and Statistical Manual of Mental Disorders* (*DSM-III*, American Psychiatric Association 1980). This recognition coincides with prior work by the author at the National Institute of Mental Health and unequivocally includes catastrophic natural and personal events as notable and significant stressors. In concert with the formal appearance of PTSD, a program was developed to address the research, treatment, and training issues surrounding this phenomenon (Frederick 1977b). For example, the Disaster Relief Act of 1974, PL 93-288, section 413, specifically addresses the crisis-counseling and training

I thank Denise Paz for her assistance with the statistical analysis of the data.

aspects of disastrous events (*Federal Register* 1976). To receive this assistance are children and adults in geographically stricken areas of disaster. Definitive rules and regulations governing the implementation of that act were developed by the author in cooperation with the Federal Disaster Assistance Administration, now the Federal Emergency Management Agency (FEMA). The Disaster Relief Act itself has focused primarily upon natural disasters as opposed to human-induced events, although federal aid is available for any catastrophic event affecting a large number of people when it is beyond the scope of local management to handle it.

In the federal regulations governing the use of government funds to ameliorate disastrous consequences, *major disaster* is defined to mean

> any hurricane, tornado, storm, flood, high water, wind-driven water, tidal wave, tsunami, earthquake, volcanic eruption, landslide, mudslide, snow storm, drought, fire, explosion, or *other catastrophe* [emphasis added] in any part of the United States which, in the determination of the President, causes damage of sufficient severity and magnitude to warrant major disaster assistance under the Act (Public Law 93-288) above and beyond emergency services by the Federal Government to supplement the efforts and available resources of the States, local governments, and disaster relief organizations, in alleviating the damage, loss, hardship, or suffering caused thereby.

Provision is made inherent in these regulations to render needed services for any type of catastrophic situation that exceeds the state's capability for management. In the context, of PL 93-288, *crisis* means "the existence of any life situations resulting from a major disaster or its aftermath which so affects the emotional and mental equilibrium of a disaster victim that professional mental health counseling services should be provided to help preclude possible damaging physical or psychological effects." In order to maintain standards and provide service at an appropriate level, *disaster workers* are defined to mean "mental health specialists such as psychiatrists, psychologists, psychiatric nurses, social workers or qualified agents thereof." Not only is allowance made for providing needed services to victims in the immediate disaster situation but for its *aftermath* as well. This recognition served as a precursor to and predated the printing of post-traumatic stress disorders in *DSM-III*. The regulations noted were written by the author and approved by the Public Health Service/National Institute of Mental Health and printed in the Federal Register on November 26, 1976. Specifically with regard to children, some of the early references to the effects of psychic trauma are made in the professional literature, discussing tornadoes, Bloch et al. (1953); regarding floods, Newman (1976); on floods, earthquakes, and tornadoes, Frederick (1977a), and Cullen and Connolly (1982); and discussing political siege, McWhirter and Trew (1982). At the outset it is important to note a list of common psychiatric disturbances found among children (shown in Table 1).

Deleterious physical or psychological effects can occur when stressors are put on children directly or are suffered by their parents. This has been observed in nonhumans in measuring the effects of prenatal maternal stress upon the behavior of rat offspring (Thompson et al. 1962). Three types of stressors were studied separately, including conditioned anxiety. An anxiety-provoking signal was given three times daily to pregnant mothers with the instrumental-avoidance response being blocked. Offspring showed significant differences in activity levels, latency of anxiety, frequency of defecation, and in learning to traverse a runway. These behavioral symptoms were present more than four months later, although less marked than at one month. It is apparent that stressors affect maternal physiology, which in turn affects the offspring. Illustratively, adrenalectomy in pregnant mothers produces hypertrophy of the fetal adrenal glands (Ingle and Fisher 1938). Increasing dosages of adrenocorticotrophic hormone (ACTH) given to the mother results in alterations in fetal cholesterol and depletion of fetal adrenal ascorbic acid (Jones et al. 1953; Josimovich et al. 1954).

At the human level, investigators (Hall et al. 1982) have observed that women who have experienced emotional stress have more difficult pregnancies and deliveries than women who do not experience such stress. They note further that stressful experiences in human mothers as well as nonhuman mothers affect activity level, birth weight, heart rate, motor development, and emotionality of the offspring.

Moreover, it has been noted that when pregnant women experience a variety of emotions, including sudden grief, fear, or anxiety, this invariably causes violent activity on the part of the fetuses (Sontag 1966). In one instance, when a woman's husband threatened to kill her, the fetus kicked so violently that it evoked extreme pain in the mother. Recordings following this incident showed a 10-fold increase in activity over the levels previously checked during weekly examinations. After the babies studied by Sontag were born, they were irritable, extremely hyperactive, and in some instances displayed severe feeding problems. While the effects of prenatal PTSD in mothers, per se, has not been studied, it is not unlikely that severe cases can affect offspring in pre- and postnatal periods.

Table 1. Common Psychiatric Disturbances Found Among Children in Selected Catastrophic Situations, in Relative Frequency of Occurrences

	Disasters		Child Molestation		Physical Abuse
Rank	DSM-III Disorder	Rank	DSM-III Disorder	Rank	DSM-III Disorder
1	313.21 Anxiety disorder, avoidant disorder	1	308.20 Post-traumatic stress disorder, acute	1	313.00 Overanxious disorder
2	309.12 Anxiety disorder, separation-anxiety disorder	2	309.81 Post-traumatic stress disorder chronic	2	313.21 Anxiety disorder, avoidant disorder
3	307.46 Sleep-terror disorder	3	300.29 Simple phobia	3	307.46 Sleep-terror disorder
4	313.00 Overanxious disorder	4	313.82 Identity disorder	4	308.20 Post-traumatic stress disorder, acute
5	300.29 Simple phobia	5	313.81 Oppositional disorder	5	309.81 Post-traumatic stress disorder, chronic
6	300.22 Agoraphobia, without panic	6	300.02 Generalized anxiety disorder	6	309.40 Adjustment disorder
7	308.20 Post-traumatic stress disorder, acute	7	309.24 Adjustment disorder with anxious mood	7	314.01 Attention-deficit disorder, with hyperactivity
8	309.81 Post-traumatic stress disorder, chronic	8	300.81 Somatization disorder	8	300.29 Simple phobia
9	314.01 Attention-deficit disorder with hyperactivity	9	300.22 Agoraphobia without panic	9	305.00 Functional enuresis
10	314.80 Attention-deficit disorder, residual type	10	309.00 Adjustment disorder, residual type	10	313.82 Identity disorder

Short-Term Effects

The most common psychological and behavioral symptoms manifest in children across all disastrous events, in the short-run, are these: sleep disorders (bad dreams), persistent thoughts of the trauma, belief that another traumatic event will occur, conduct disturbances, hyperalertness, avoidance of any stimulus or situation symbolic of the event, psychophysiological disturbances, and, in younger children, regression to enuresis, thumbsucking, and more-dependent behavior. Some of these may continue into long-term symptoms.

The contagious effects of psychic trauma on children when parental figures or surrogates are affected must not be underestimated. These phenomena have been observed in a variety of traumatic situations due to parental anxieties, fears, tensions, and apprehension. Children may become exceptionally upset because the usually stalwart figures in their lives are perceived as being unstable. This phenomenon was observed in World War II in England when parental fears precipitated more emotional difficulty for the children than the explosion of bombs (Freud and Burlingham 1943). Parental instability can lead to world-destruction fantasies in very young children, because a child's world collapses when the most stable objects in it lack solidity. This has been especially apparent when such fears are augmented by a catastrophic event outside the home situation, for example during the San Fernando Valley earthquake in 1971 (Howard and Gordon 1972).Children developed dramatic forms of separation anxiety, manifested by clinging to parents, hiding under beds, and refusing to go to school. A mutually infectious contagion developed from child to parent and parent to child as a result of this deleterious interactive process.

While the behavior of children at Three Mile Island (TMI) has not been studied fully as yet, the mothers of young children were at high risk for experiencing clinical episodes of anxiety and depression during the year following the event (Bromet 1980). Such clinical episodes were not associated with other forms of stress or support factors and therefore were related solely to that traumatic event. In particular, these mothers reported more symptoms of anxiety and depression at subclinical levels during interviews, compared with mothers at a companion nuclear site in western Pennsylvania. In other words, symptoms were present which had not evoked entry into any mental health system. Nevertheless, it is apparent that the accident affected a sizable number of people.

Figure 1 shows the high percentage of children involved in the evacuation, from among some 34,000 persons living within a five-

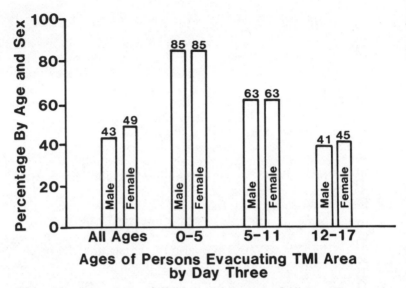

Figure 1. Percentages of Children and Persons of All Ages Evacuated at Three Mile Island by the Third Day after the Accident, Arranged by Age and Sex (Adapted from Goldhaber MK, Lehman JE: Crisis evacuation during the Three Mile Island nuclear accident: the TMI population registry, presented at the 1982 annual meeting of the American Public Health Association, held in Montreal)

mile radius of the plant. Persons with the greatest symptoms of distress were those who lived within a five-mile radius of the plant, had less-adequate social support from friends and relatives, and those who had some prior history of mental health or emotional disturbance, although that is not a requisite for the presence of PTSD. Being pregnant at the time of the accident was also a high-risk factor. The physical or mental health effects of radiation dose levels of a few rems or less are not fully known. Estimates of the potential health effects of the TMI accident are based on extrapolations from the known health effects of higher levels of radiation. Effects from the actual amounts received at TMI appear to be virtually nonexistent. The average likely dose of actual radiation that any person received was less than 100 millirems (less than that in two or three chest x-rays) (Upton 1981; Gur et al. 1983). Symptoms of distress resembling PTSD criteria were found in students living within a five-mile radius of the plant and among those with a preschool sibling (Dohrenwend et al. 1981).

Thus, the major health effect of the accident appears to have been upon the mental health of the people living in the region of Three Mile Island and of the workers at the plant. There was immediate, short-lived mental distress produced by the accident among certain groups of the general population living within 20 miles of TMI. The highest levels of distress were found among adults, (*a*) living within 5 miles of TMI, or (*b*) with preschool children; and among teenagers, (*a*) living within 5 miles of TMI, (*b*) with preschool siblings, or (*c*) whose families left the area. Workers at TMI experienced more distress than workers at another plant, operating normally at the time, in western Pennsylvania that was studied for comparison purposes. This distress was higher among the nonsupervisory employees, and continued in the months following the accident.

Long-Term Effects

The long-term and post-traumatic impact of disasters has been observed repeatedly by the author in numerous catastrophes (Frederick 1983). A recent study of the psychological impact of the Mount St. Helens volcano disclosed that domestic violence increased 46 percent and stress-aggravated illness 198 percent at the end of the seven-month period following the disaster (Adams and Adams 1984). Moreover, there was an increase of 236 percent in the monthly average of mental illness cases and of 219 percent in psychosomatic illness. These marked increases were manifest in children and adults alike with neither standing out as being more prone to distress than the other. These results compared both pre- and postdisaster base lines on objective, community-based statistical data. The assumption was that stress-related problems would be manifested in the observable and recorded behavior of disaster victims. This study relied upon empirical data rather than clinical anecdotal impressions. Although there were decreases in child abuse and divorce, of 89 percent and 6 percent, respectively, the increase of 46 percent in domestic violence is particularly significant. Among children, increases occurred in juvenile criminal bookings of 2½ percent; vandalism/malicious mischief, 24 percent; and charges of disorderly conduct, 10 percent. Each of these showed substantial increases over the base-line data obtained for the four months prior to the volcanic eruption. In essence then, traumatic psychological and behavioral reactions affected much of the population, including children (personal communication from Adams and Adams 1984). Significantly, it should be emphasized that these reactions were not of a transient nature, since they obtained at a point seven months following the traumatic event.

During the severe winter storms and flooding in Boston in 1977 it was reported that high school youngsters in physical education classes displayed a marked increase in blood pressure (Cohen and Ahearn 1980). These phenomena were clearly correlated with the stress related to that catastrophic event and abated when crisis-intervention services were provided and the conditions associated with family stress were ameliorated.

At a follow-up, on-site visit, seven months after the devastating tornado in Xenia, Ohio, in April 1974, the author met with four prominent citizens representing that community, two men and two women, so as to evaluate the area's existing health needs. All of them expressed their views, and vividly described their experiences during and after the tornado. In doing so, each victim wept openly, revealing the tenuous quality of their efforts toward repression and problem resolution. It was clear that none of these people had experienced any form of deconditioning or of working through the trauma, which had become imprinted in their psyches. The psychological marks made upon children were detailed, including accounts of how sharing classrooms in other schools and functioning in temporary locations brought intolerable stresses to bear upon both teachers and students. Crowded conditions evoked perceptions of encroachment so that the displaced students from other schools were seen as interlopers. Tensions and annoyances mounted, with the result that students developed conduct problems and psychophysiological disorders, while truancy increased. Teachers quit speaking to each other. Symptoms of PTSD were clearly in evidence among the adult and childhood populations in Xenia. With appropriate and timely intervention such problems could have been readily avoided.

In the Buffalo Creek Dam disaster in 1972, which was a calamity containing both natural and human-induced factors, 125 people were killed, most of whom were women and children. Many child survivors saw others drown, or viewed frightening sights of blood and gore. Still others who did not see these aspects of the disaster suffered because of their parents' inability to reconstruct their own lives. This evoked long-term effects upon the children. In a legal suit evolving from the Buffalo Creek disaster, attorneys documented the fact that 226 children received a total of two million dollars for mental suffering, which was put into a trust fund, with each to receive his or her share at age 18 (Stern 1976).

Worthy of note are Erikson's (1976) and Newman's (1976) singularly important works regarding adult and child victims at Buffalo Creek. Astute observations were made about the loss of communality among the members of that population, at both group and individual level. The social fabric of the community was broken by the upheaval and displacement. A marked increase in the use of alcohol and drugs developed, as well as thefts; these served as an index of the social disorganization. Perhaps the cruelest cut of all was the young people who seemed to be slipping away from the control of parents and were involved in nameless delinquencies. In a culture that was traditionally concerned about the continuity between generations this is particularly distressing, and connotes certain aspects of PTSD, when accompanied by the other symptoms of a mental health nature. Although overt psychic numbing is seen in adults, among children and adolescents it often takes the form of withdrawal into uncustomary behavioral patterns. Children under 12 years of age were studied through a description of their responses in terms of unusual fantasies, vulnerability to future stress, an altered sense of power over the self, and an early awareness of fragmentation and death (Newman 1976). It was noted that these factors can lead to subsequent trauma later in life when an effective adaptation is not made through appropriate treatment. The effects of the disaster were attributed to three main factors: (1) developmental level at the time of the trauma, (2) the children's perceptions of reactions in the family to the catastrophic event, and (3) direct exposure of the children themselves to the trauma. Phobic reactions, sleep difficulties, and anxieties about symbolic events were clearly those of PTSD experienced by children.

COMPARISONS OF STRESSFUL EVENTS— CHILDREN AND ADULTS

Many of these same responses were observed in child victims by the author and his colleagues when providing intervention following a sniper shooting at a school yard in Los Angeles where 15 persons were shot and 1 young girl died at the site. The assailant, himself, suffered from PTSD, which had stemmed from the deaths of his parents and some siblings in the Jonestown massacre in Guyana. The psychological autopsy performed by the author on the assailant disclosed both acute and chronic traumatic effects brought about by Jonestown while the assailant was in his late teens. Further data pertaining to that psychological autopsy, as well as to PTSD in the children who were victims of the event, are being developed and prepared in separate studies by the author.

From 300 cases of child molestation studied by the author, 30 are reported herein, with regard to specific responses to a Reaction Index (PTSD scale) the author has employed to study victims of a variety of extreme stressors, including natural disasters, human-induced catastrophic events, physical abuse, assault, and child molestation. These data have also been studied in the adult population to include, in addition to the types of cases noted above, persons who have been held hostage, physically battered, raped, or have witnessed the violent death of a loved one. If some form of violence accompanies the traumatic event the likelihood of a severe psychological reaction is usually increased. In the author's experience, victims of violently intrusive events are particularly prone to experience PTSD with long-term psychological problems. Moreover, when a child is above school age and likely to be more fully cognizant of the circumstances, the psychological sequelae may be more severe. Among some 300 cases of child molestation, the author has never seen any case beyond the age of six where PTSD was not in evidence. Feelings of loss of self-control and power over one's personal environment are critical. Such psychic trauma can be triggered by a variety of stressors (e.g., the turbulence involved in a natural disaster—earthquakes, floods, or tornadoes; sexual abuse; being held hostage; or witnessing a violent death.

Victims characteristically engage in conscious and unconscious attempts to manage the stress. Studies of Israeli children who were exposed to bombings were compared with other youngsters in towns where no shellings had occurred. Exposed children required more sleep, day dreamed less, and were more compromising toward the Arabs than were unexposed subjects (Ziv et al. 1974; Rofe and Lewin 1980). The results indicated that communal and adult support and reassurance were important in bringing about adjustment. However, the concept of the *return of the repressed*, so to speak, does seem to appear later, in exposed children. The concept of latent traumatic neurotic responses in youngsters 10–12 years of age living in the Jordan valley was studied 2 years after exposure to bombings, and it was found that the youngsters who were shelled manifested bruxism, especially during sleep, and psychophysiologic conditions associated with tension (Kristal 1978). Youngsters who had been exposed to shellings reported higher anxiety levels when watching stressful films associated with terrorist attacks than their nonshelled peers. These results obtained even though anxiety levels were similar in neutral or nonsymbolically traumatic situations. This is consonant with some of the differences appearing between youngsters and adults with respect to PTSD symptoms.

The Reaction Index or PTSD scale was standardized in 750 childhood cases and 1350 adult cases of stress-laden events. The correlation with established cases of PTSD among children was .91, and .95 among adults. An earlier version (Laube and Murphy 1985) has now been updated, and includes a five-point scale with item ratings

Table 2. Post-Traumatic Stress Disorder in Children Experiencing
Different Types of Traumatic Events

	N	Observed	Expected
Disasters	50	30	10
Child molestation	50	50	10
Physical abuse	50	35	10
Total	150	115	30
Disasters	$\chi^2 = 15.04$	$df = 1$	$p = .0001$
Child molestation	$\chi^2 = 63.37$	$df = 1$	$p = .0001$
Physical abuse	$\chi^2 = 23.27$	$df = 1$	$p = .0001$
All forms of trauma	$\chi^2 = 94.18$	$df = 1$	$p = .0001$

from *None of the Time* to *Most of the Time*. The items specify reactions
described in *DSM-III* and may be given vicariously if necessary.
Scoring ranges from 0 to 4 for each item with a total of 80 possible
points. Some items are phrased in reverse order so that scoring is
not always in the same direction. Degrees of severity range from
Doubtful, when the score is less than 12, to *Very Severe*, when the
score is greater than 60.

In the data reported here 150 children (less than 18 years of age)
were studied, covering three areas of stress; disasters, child molestation, and physical abuse, with 50 subjects in each group. For comparison, 350 adults cases are also cited, covering the following stressors: natural disasters; human-induced catastrophes (e.g., aircraft
accidents, bombings, auto accidents with injury, industrial accidents,
and witnessing violent deaths); hostages; and physical battering/
assault. Although not included for our purpose in the present treatise,
military combat cases were also incorporated into the original total
sample. The cases presented in this article showed both acute and
chronic, or delayed, symptoms of PTSD. The sample populations
reported came from persons seen at helping agencies, legal services
both public and private, and personal referral, and thus came from
a common population of help-seeking victims of intrusive stressors.
In the total original/experimental sample, the Reaction Index was
administered to every other case seen and compared with controls
from the general population comprised of persons seen in helping
agencies, hospitals, clinics, and universities for reasons other than
mental conditions. The data clearly reveal marked cases of PTSD

Table 3. Post-Traumatic Stress Disorders in Adults Experiencing Different Types of Traumatic Events

	N	Observed	Expected
Natural disasters	100	40	20
Human-induced catastrophes	50	25	10
Hostages	100	68	20
Physical assault	100	65	20
Total	350	198	70
Natural disasters	$\chi^2 = 8.59$	$df = 1$	$p = .003$
Human-induced catastrophes	$\chi^2 = 8.61$	$df = 1$	$p = .003$
Hostages	$\chi^2 = 44.82$	$df = 1$	$p = .0001$
Physical assault	$\chi^2 = 39.61$	$df = 1$	$p = .0001$
All forms of trauma	$\chi^2 = 34.90$	$df = 1$	$p = .0001$

among all stressors shown. Table 2 discloses the significance of the three stressors noted above where the observed figures exceed those expected by highly significant levels of statistical confidence. The expected frequencies were based upon empirical clinical findings in catastrophic events wherein evidence of emotional disturbances of some kind ranged from 12 to 25 percent of the cases reporting (Tyhurst 1951; Glass 1959; Frederick 1983). Since PTSD comprises only one of a number of discernible psychological disorders reported, it constitutes a conservative base-line estimate to attribute 20 percent of the expected cases to PTSD, per se. Hence, the data are all the more striking.

Chi squares, using Yates's correction, were all statistically significant, as the reader may see from Tables 2 and 3. Significant findings obtained for the totals and for each traumatic event as well. In the children's sample, child molestation and physical abuse showed the highest figures, although disasters also surpassed chance by a large margin. Among 300 child molestation subjects examined, the author has never seen a case where symptoms of PTSD were not present in the molested if the child was over six years of age. Anxieties and withdrawal were manifest in very young children, roughly in accordance with the extent to which violence was present. With the adult population, being a hostage or the victim of physical assault, that is, victims of violent crime, appear to present a greater frequency of significant cases. Although not included in the statistical data for this article, degree of severity for PTSD victims does seem to correlate highly with chronic and delayed symptoms as well. Table 4 reveals a strong difference between adult and child victims in favor of the latter. Of child victims, 77 percent presented PTSD, compared with 57 percent of the adults. Similar results have been found for children exposed to the traumatic event of being taken hostage (Van der Ploeg 1983; Terr 1981). It is clear that some differences in precise criteria evolve in children when compared with adults. The appearance of psychic numbing, in particular, appears in another form or is not obvious. Children are likely to manifest unique avoidance behaviors as a form of numbing. For example, they may initially draw a picture of something other than the catastrophic event, or avoid using a coloring book when other children are doing so and become less verbal than they were prior to the event.

Personality profiles on the Minnesota Multiphasic Personality Inventory (MMPI) have been obtained for older children and adults following traumatic events, such as those noted, with stressors which activate PTSDs, as listed in *DSM-III*. These cases were gathered from a variety of events including floods, tornadoes, physical assaults (sexual abuse and battering) in the child (adolescent) population, $N = 48$. While these numbers are selectively small they do seem to be indicative of a persistent phenomenon heretofore unreported. Work with young Viet Nam veterans confirms these findings on the MMPI in that population (Fairbank et al. 1983). Preliminary findings on PTSD scales developed by the author for children as well as adults have correlated with these findings on the MMPI. The striking similarity in configuration among adults and older children is revealed in Figure 2. The relatively high F scale with respect to the K scale is indicative of the acute quality of the PTSD disturbance and does not suggest malingering. The peak on the left side of the profile is in keeping

Table 4. Incidence of PTSD in Adults and Children Experiencing Different Traumas

	Adult (57%)	Child (77%)	Total
Yes	198	115	313
No	152	35	187
Total	350	150	500

Note. $\chi^2 = 17.26$; $df = 1$; $p = .0001$.

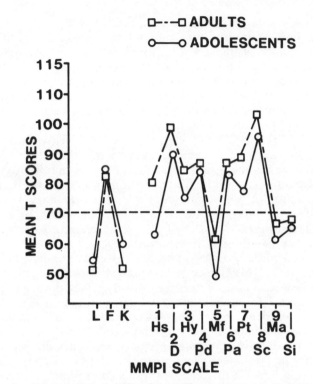

Figure 2. Typical Case Profile of the Effects of Stress in Post-Traumatic Stress Disorder Found in Adults and Late Adolescents

with heightened anxiety and/or feelings of depression, while the peak on the right side of the profile denotes the impact of the trauma upon thinking and perception. Its intensity reaches heights so marked as to border on irrationality. The low points indicate that such persons are sitting on an emotional lid, so to speak, attempting to hold acting-out tendencies in abeyance. The marked low valley in the profile at Mf is associated with sexual self-concept and can suggest an effort to reassure oneself of one's basic masculinity or femininity under stress, depending upon the sex. It may also indicate that although other parts of the personality pattern may change with stress basic self-concept usually remains intact, even in persons who may attempt to simulate more serious disturbances than they actually have (as suggested by Dr. Martin Symonds [personal communication]). Irritability, rebellion, and suspiciousness are disclosed in the peaks at Pd and Pa.

Salient Questions

What reactions are likely to occur in children in particular from catastrophic situations? Responses are apt to cover at least two spheres, chiefly those which encompass behavioral and emotional reactions. As the reader may note from Table 1, a variety of psychiatric disturbances may occur which require intervention. Particularly prominent are those affecting young children which need direct physical support in contradistinction to the symptoms which appear among adults. Of course, all age groups affected will require appropriate diagnostic and treatment services. By being alert and sensitive to the probability that sleep disturbances will occur, both parents and professional persons alike can take steps necessary to effect an amelioration of these traumatic effects.

Where and when are disorders likely to occur? The most likely areas in the youngster's life where disturbances will appear are at home or at school. Sleep disorders often appear almost immediately, behavior problems usually surface later. This is why both parents and teachers should watch for any change in behavior which continues for more than a week or two. Disturbances at home are more apt to involve conduct problems and sleep disorders, which can translate into the school setting as the problems develop at home. Sleep disorders may reveal themselves to alert teachers in the form of apathy, weariness, loss of concentration, and irritability, somewhat later. Appropriate referral can then be made. Young children may reveal separation anxiety almost immediately, along with sleep disturbances. Misconduct often comes into the picture after a few weeks of enduring the stresses accompanying the traumatic event.

CONSIDERATIONS FOR INTERVENTION

Depending upon the age of the child various forms of therapeutic interventions are in order in times of crisis. Younger children, in particular, even under ordinary circumstances, do not have the verbal skills to fully express their tensions and fears. Even adults, in periods of extreme stress and crisis, do not possess the verbal skills ordinarily within their command. With children, then, it is necessary to utilize nonverbal means both to observe problems and to treat them when they occur.

Signs to Recognize

1. Sleep disturbances that continue for more than several days, wherein actual dreams of the trauma may or may not appear.
2. Separation anxiety or clinging behavior, such as a reluctance to return to school.

3. Phobias about distressing stimuli (e.g., a school building, TV scene, or person) that remind the victim of the traumatic event.
4. Conduct disturbances, including problems that occur at home or at school, which serve as responses to anxiety and frustration.
5. Doubts about the self, including comments about body confusion, self-worth, and desire for withdrawal.

Children are apprehensive about being separated from the stable guideposts of their family environment and are equally fearful that the catastrophic event will recur. It is important for parents and teachers to anticipate such fears and be prepared to address them. Any major unsettling or traumatic event will usually evoke a fear response. This is not abnormal behavior, in and of itself, but it must be recognized and dealt with in order to preclude the possibility of more serious sequelae later.

It is to be expected that adults, including parents and teachers, will breathe a sigh of relief, psychologically as well as physically, after a calamitous event and feel that problems are past. Once the impact of the event is over persons tend to count their blessings and become imbued with the thought that everything of an unsettling nature is past. Nothing could be further from the truth. Because of the need to dismiss unpleasant events from their own thoughts, adults may not be alert or responsive to signs of distress in children. Emotional reactions still present in children as well as adults are precursors to PTSD and other problems of an emotional and mental health nature, which must be addressed.

EFFECTS OF TRAUMA AND SYMPTOMS UPON TREATMENT AND PROGNOSIS

The trauma itself has direct and indirect, or symbolic, representation in environmental stimuli. The traumatic stressor may be a person or a situation. When it recurs, even symbolically, avoidance ensues, in effect to diminish the subjective negative feelings. Thus, prognosis becomes less positive as well. When violence is involved, the severity of the trauma affects one's ability to form therapeutic alliances or relate readily to a treatment effort. A difficulty in coping with aggression develops since the anger is directed inwardly toward the already damaged and fear-laden self. In general, the more severe the trauma the greater the fear. Psychic severity is in the eye of the beholder. Those who actually see physical trauma fear lack of control over their own lives and become silent and uncommunicative; hence, they are often overlooked and go untreated. Children who live with its effects upon significant others can be negatively affected, as indicated in survivors of the Nazi holocaust (Danieli 1981a, b; 1985).

The symptoms displayed affect treatment and prognosis. The symptom patterns discussed are not unique to youngsters in the United States. Prominent symptoms (e.g., phobias, nightmares, and psychophysiological reactions) found by the author (Frederick 1983) have also been reported in Europe (Van der Ploeg 1983). In a sample of youngsters held hostage in a school in the Netherlands, more than one-third developed phobias, 32 percent showed insomnia and 41 percent revealed tension. The latter resembled the psychophysiological symptoms of increased blood pressure and stomach problems found by the author. These symptoms all necessitate focused attention upon them in treatment. Favorable prognosis is lessened by lack of treatment and length of time given to specific facets of the problem. The longer symptoms continue, treated or untreated, the poorer the prognosis. When PTSD is present but missed, which is a frequent occurrence in younger age groups, inappropriate treatment is given, if any at all.

Children remember basic sensory stimuli, such as sounds or colors, in traumatic situations. Cognitive confusion occurs in perception. Children will recall the awesome sounds and colors of a tornado, the rumble and rattling of an earthquake, shots from the gunfire of police or others, olfactory stimuli from debris, or the closeness of crowded living conditions. These more-primitive responses overwhelm the egos of children since, many of such usual adult defense mechanisms as intellectualization, rationalization, and denial have not developed in prepubescent children.

The victim can, and often does, become a victimizer. Sexually molested children tend to molest others. Children who are physically abused are apt to become abusers. Albert De Salvo, the Boston Strangler, stated that he was beaten with a belt every night, whether he misbehaved or not. Consonant with the traumatic incidents that have evoked serious mental and emotional problems, especially PTSD, victims frequently become suicidal and self-destructive in their behavior. Suicide ranks among the first 10 leading causes of death in adults, and third in persons under the age of 20. However, it is the first leading cause of unnecessary deaths. No one should die by suicide if they have an effective therapeutic relationship. This is not to say that persons do not take their lives while in psychotherapy but, invariably, when it occurs, something has been missing in the therapy. The pain and anguish evoking such behavior simply have not been reached or dealt with when such tragic behavior occurs. From the author's experience as a former president of the American Association of Suicidology and director of an NIMH program in suicide prevention, repeated evidence for this has been apparent. It is a particularly regrettable and tragic phenomenon when it occurs in young people who have not really begun to live their lives. There is no guarantee, of course, that any procedure will always prevent the act, but all suicides are unnecessary deaths and every therapist who works with victims should be trained in suicide prevention. It cannot and should not be viewed in the same light as death from a terminal disease or serious accident, resulting from gross force.

TREATMENT TECHNIQUES

A variety of techniques have been used in catastrophic situations with children as well as with adults. A requisite for all of these is the creation of an environment which is safe where a supportive figure is present. This creates a climate where traumatic feelings can be reworked, permitting the ultimate reduction of debilitating anxiety. Some techniques employed with children follow.

The Coloring Storybook

This method was used by mental health workers following a tornado in Omaha, Nebraska in 1975. The coloring book should be one which describes the traumatic event, and is given to the child to color with the request that the child relate it to himself or herself. The instructions should be given to both teachers and parents, pointing out that it is not unusual to feel anxious and uncomfortable following the traumatic event. It is also important not to transmit one's own uncertainties, and to provide support to the children as needed. Parents and teachers are reminded that although children may have difficulty expressing themselves in order to overcome bad memories and fears, using a coloring book can facilitate that procedure. It should be emphasized that it is important for the parent and teacher to let children know they are loved and that they are not alone. Children must be encouraged to write down even their fearful thoughts, and they ought to be helped to know that other youngsters have also been afraid. The material should describe the traumatic event as such. For example, a page might define a tornado by talking about rain and cold and hot air coming together. Another page can emphasize the fact that nobody can stop a tornado once it begins. A house may be pictured, with instructions for youngsters to go to a safe area such as a basement and listen for warning signals. Then the child is asked to draw a tornado (or applicable trauma event) and tell what he or she did when the tornado came and what happened afterward. In this way, the youngster can begin a catharsis and experience some desensitization to the ongoing fears.

Drawings

Structured. A structured drawing is one in which the child is told what to draw. For example, the child might be instructed to draw his or her house at the time of a tornado or earthquake and to put significant beings in the drawing, such as members of one's own family or pets. This has the advantage of eliciting specific responses that relate directly to the event while minimizing the likelihood of getting material which may not relate to the trauma itself.

Unstructured. An unstructured drawing is one in which the child is given little or no instruction about what to draw. Youngsters may be told to draw whatever they feel is important or would like to draw. Some children may be hesitant to draw aspects of the traumatic event which they have suffered, at the first attempt. In this case, they are permitted to draw something else, which may not be at the same level of consciousness in terms of any anxiety attached to the event as such. In so doing, a second drawing, after the first, can elicit material about the traumatic event more easily. It has been observed that sometimes a youngster will draw a picture that is partially related to the event but does not directly describe it or involve the child, per se. In most instances, however, children will produce a drawing about the traumatic event when encouraged to do so in a supportive manner. For therapeutic and diagnostic purposes it is important to help the child reach the point where a drawing can be rendered which is related to the catastrophic situation. If this is not done, then the fears surrounding it will not be worked through and will continue to plague the child. For example, profitable drawings were elicited by Newman after the Buffalo Creek Dam disaster in 1972, in West Virginia (Newman 1976)

Instruction Booklets

An instruction booklet developed by workers at the San Fernando Valley earthquake in 1971 and published in 1973 focused upon information of use to both adults and children, although with young children, emphasis was placed first upon working with the adult rather than dealing with the child directly.

Play Therapy

Most experienced therapists find play therapy of use with young children because it helps in the communication of fears without placing importance upon verbal skills. It also enables the therapist to arrange material in a planned fashion by introducing significant figures and events for therapeutic use. A backdrop can be established, both figuratively and literally, against which to play out scenes involving the child's emotional difficulties. Important surrogate figures and the child's own feelings can be brought into focus in an effective manner by a skilled and understanding psychotherapist. This procedure has been advocated by mental health clinicians, stemming from the Nicaraguan earthquake in 1972 (Cohen and Ahearn 1980).

Group Psychotherapy

Group psychotherapy may be of some value, especially in conjunction with other activities. A specific form of it may be used in a classroom, while evoking discussion about drawings that have been produced by the youngsters. This is likely to be of more value for youngsters who are eight years of age or older. They are apt to interact with each other in group discussions more readily than younger children, who are more likely to play alongside each other rather than with each other. Support can come from hearing other youngsters talk about their own fears. The notion of being afraid or feeling "silly" is normalized and universalized, so to speak, in a situation of this type. It is important to ask each child what happened and what his or her fears were. It is useful to discuss any specific stories which may have developed and to provide factual information in order to disavow misbeliefs which may been engendered. Rumors about events which did not occur will often add to the stress and needlessly heighten the problems at hand.

Incident-Specific Treatment

When severe PTSD is in evidence, in contrast to avoidant anxiety states or other diagnostic entities, it is necessary to invoke incident-specific treatment, individually tailored and based upon relearning. While this procedure may be utilized by skillful trained therapists through several methods (e.g., play therapy or group psychotherapy), the author has usually found it most fruitful to employ it in individual sessions. Treatment specific to the trauma has been widely employed with adult victims as well. In the author's experience, it is the only procedure that resolves severe cases of PTSD. It customarily encompasses a frame-by-frame, slow-motion reworking process. It is our firm view that this process is a sine qua non for the effective management of any severe psychic trauma. This is especially true where nightmares and phobic reactions are in evidence, even though they may abate somewhat after the trauma. Although many children will be troubled and display school-avoidant problems following a disastrous event, only those who are seriously distressed will continue to manifest this behavior for more than a couple of weeks. It is of paramount importance to provide parents and after-school authorities with appropriate information in order to enlist their cooperation and support for diagnostic screening and an initial therapeutic effort in these settings. Moreover, some subjects will at least partially repress the trauma, only to have it reappear later.

Where possible, it is of particular value to return the subject to the location where he or she was at the time of the catastrophe. This process is appropriate for both adults and children. Thus, if the youngster was at school it may be of inestimable value to recreate the scene in the school setting under skilled direction. If a child was at home or another place which is readily accessible, then, where possible, it may be most useful in undoing the trauma to place the child back in that setting while providing support and helping the child to work through the difficulty. If the youngster was in a particular room at home at the time of the event it may be helpful to recapture the actual scene associated with the trauma. This can be done, literally in vivo and/or through imagery, "in vitro," by reestablishing the scene in the mind of the young victim. Merely talking or "rapping" will not suffice in undoing serious psychic trauma in either adults or children. *Trauma mastery must be incident-specific for specific resolution of the problem.* Caveats must be emphasized here, to caution persons against moving too abruptly into incident-specific replays, on the one hand, and avoiding any focus upon them, on the other. This procedure should not be confused with behavior modification nor is it synonymous with the technique of flooding. Relaxation prior to the process enables the stressors to be tolerated and accepted for relearning purposes. Much care and sensitivity are required to delineate debilitating psychic traumas. Feelings surrounding them are carefully explored for generalization to other aspects of life.

Unfortunately, the author has encountered many cases of traumatic situations, particularly among adults, where the victim has undergone treatment for years without effective resolution of the trauma, because of inadequate and misguided therapeutic endeavors that did not focus upon the central aspects of the trauma. Children as well as adults are apt to be confused about their fears and anxiety states. The confusion stems not only from misconceptions that have surrounded the event itself but from a lack of understanding of, and doubt about, the nature of their feelings and the fact that these feelings have evolved in a systematic and logical way. They should be helped to undo the doubts and experience these feelings directly. Victims must realize that they are not abnormal for experiencing turbulent emotional responses, since a sizable number of other persons of their age levels have similar feelings in similar situations. *Universalizing* the experience helps to reduce anxiety and provide the support needed under such stressful conditions. Individually tailored stimulus and response procedures must be used to diminish and extinguish distressing reactions.

Following the San Fernando earthquake in 1971, the author provided consultation to workers at the San Fernando Valley Child Guidance Clinic and facilitated grant support for a small NIMH study to examine the effects of crisis counseling in that calamity. Within a few days after the earthquake, hundreds of calls were received by various agencies, including those at the San Fernando Clinic. Displaying separation-anxiety, children clung to their parents and feared returning to school as a consequence of that tragic temblor. Underscoring the need to provide *psychological immunization*, as the author termed it at the time, it was apparent that desensitizing the children's fears was the order of the day. It was recommended that various dimensions of the earthquake be relived by showing slides and scenes of other quakes, by role playing what individuals did and what they might do if the temblor were to occur again. The importance of addressing particularly frightening scenes was emphasized. Support of family and friends, and personal responsibility were also underscored. Specific aspects of the program, recommended to the clinic for its victims at that time, have been employed on a wide scale since, especially vis-à-vis incident-specific refocusing procedures. In such events it is necessary to create an "in vitro" situation simulating an in vivo one in order to rework and undo the victim's fears. Intervention procedures were effective for victims served.

The following outline should be of value for those who work with both children and adults in severe post-traumatic situations. It is adapted from a government publication edited by the author (Frederick 1981) when dealing with aircraft accidents.

Outline of Specific Requirements for Key Workers in Major Emergency Situations with Adults and Childhood Victims

I. Skills Needed
    A. Facility for administration where groups of victims are involved
        1. Mobilize emergency relief workers, including volunteers.
        2. Collaborate with and provide leadership for various people and organizations.

3. Provide accurate and prompt information and thereby control rumors.
4. Supply follow-up care of victims.
5. Train volunteers to provide effective emotional first aid to victims.
B. Facility for providing emotional support
  1. Relieve emotional distress.
    a. Project competence, calmness, firmness, encouragement.
    b. Maintain a nonjudgmental attitude.
    c. Provide reassurance; encourage relatives to supply physical comfort, especially for children; allow children to sleep near trusting parents on a temporary basis.
  2. Alleviate feelings of guilt—stressing the fact that self-blame and fears are not uncommon.
    d. Establish rapport; exercise empathy.
    e. Listen creatively; remain attentive; establish eye contact; convey respect and understanding for victims' experiences.
    f. Focus the problems and assist in constructive planning (e.g., help with funeral arrangements, contact victims' local community mental health centers for follow-up assistance, etc.).
    g. Reestablish and maintain hope; emphasize the resiliency of the human body and the normalcy of the emotional reactions to the intense experience.
C. Facility for recognizing emotional problems
  1. Alertness and awareness
    Mild—confused, unable to think clearly, focuses on small problems, angry, blames others
    Severe—may not give own name, date, place; has memory gaps; poor concentration
  2. Behavior
    Mild—restless, excited, agitated, still, rigid
    Severe—agitated, may perform ritualistic acts, severely depressed, withdrawn
  3. Speech
    Mild—talks rapidly, almost continually under pressure
    Severe—preoccupied with one idea or thought, may hear voices, may have delusions or avoid speaking
  4. Emotions
    Mild—cries, feelings may be blunted, inappropriately excitable, easily irritated

Severe—hard to respond or arouse, unpredictable reactions, may be hysterical

Burnout syndrome—fatigued, irritable, has impaired judgment

D. Ability to handle emotional reactions (excited, uncontrolled, or depressed responses)

1. Arrange for needed physical procedures.
2. Give instructions calmly.
3. Provide verbal reassurance.
4. Supply an authoritative attitude, expressing the expectation that orders must be followed.
5. Assign tasks for rehabilitation.

E. Facility for providing needed information.

1. Give only accurate, verified information.
2. Avoid offering false hope.
3. Impart information selectively.
4. Exercise care in accidentally imparting alarming or speculative news.
5. Scotch rumors.

II. Techniques for Developing Skills of Caregivers

A. Provide instructional lectures and supply training manuals.
B. Employ role-playing and videotape practice sessions.
C. Anticipate feelings of distress or repugnance when exposed to death and injury, and decondition personnel via exposure to hospitals, mortuaries, morgues, and by slides of injured and dead persons.
D. Expose health workers to moulage or mock injuries.
E. Use incident-specific, flooding, and/or desensitization techniques with particularly traumatic or disturbing stimuli, under skilled direction.
F. With young children, practice reliving while talking in relaxed state (e.g., accompanied by giving warm milk and reading stories).
G. Using simulations and drills where expedient.

It is hoped that the enterprising reader will be stimulated to pursue research, training, and treatment activities in this challenging area of stress disorders. While much remains to be done in the field of emergency mental health, the rewards can be immense.

REFERENCES

Adams PR, Adams GR: Mount Saint Helens's ashfall: evidence for a disaster stress reaction. Am Psychol 39:252–260, 1984

American Psychiatric Association: Diagnostic and Statistical Manual of Mental Disorders, 3rd ed. Washington, DC, American Psychiatric Association, 1980

Bloch DA, Silber E, Perry S: Some factors in the emotional reaction of child research. Washington, DC, National Academy of Sciences, 1953

Bromet E: Three Mile Island: mental health findings. (NIMH Contract No. 278-79-0048 SM), Report to the National Institute of Mental Health, 1980

Cohen RE, Ahearn FL: Handbook for Mental Health Care Victims. Baltimore, Johns Hopkins University Press, 1980

Coping with children's reaction to earthquakes and other disasters. Van Nuys, Calif, San Fernando Valley Child Guidance Clinic, 1973

Cullen J, Connolly JA: Infants under stress: tomorrow's adults, in The Child in His Family: Children in Turmoil: Tomorrow's Parents. Edited by Anthony EJ, Chiland C. New York, John Wiley & Sons, 1982

Danieli Y: Differing adaptational styles in families of survivors of the Nazi Holocaust: some implications for treatment. Child Today 10:6–10, 34–35, 1981a

Danieli Y: Families of survivors of the Nazi Holocaust: some short- and long-term effects, in Stress and Anxiety, vol. 8. Edited by Spielberger CD, Sarason IG, Milgram NA. New York, Hemisphere/McGraw-Hill, 1981b

Danieli Y: The treatment and prevention of long-term effects and intergenerational transmission of victimization: a lesson from Holocaust survivors and their children, in Trauma and Its Wake: The Study and Treatment of Post-Traumatic Stress Disorder. Edited by Figley CR. New York, Brunner/Mazel, 1985

Dohrenwend BP, Dohrenwend BS, Warheit GJ, et al: Stress in the community: a report to the President's Commission on the Accident at Three Mile Island. Annals of the New York Academy of Sciences 365:159–174, 1981

Erikson KT: Loss of communality at Buffalo Creek. Am J Psychiatry 33:302–305, 1976

Fairbank JA, Keane TM, Malloy PF: Some preliminary data on the psychological characteristics of Viet Nam veterans with post-traumatic stress disorders. J Consult Clin Psychol 6:912–919, 1983

Federal Register: Title 42 public health rules and regulations for implementation of section 413 of the Disaster Relief Act of 1974 (PL 93-288). Federal Register 41(229): Nov. 26, 1976

Frederick CJ: Current thinking about crisis or psychological intervention in U.S. disasters. Mass Emergencies 2:43–50, 1977a

Frederick CJ: Psychological first aid: emergency mental health and disaster assistance. Psychotherapy Bulletin 10:15–20, 1977b

Frederick CJ (ed): Aircraft accidents: emergency mental health problems (DHHS Publication No. ADM 81-956). Washington, DC, U.S. Government Printing Office, 1981

Frederick CJ: Violence and disaster: immediate and long-term consequences, in Helping Victims of Violence. Edited by the Ministry of Welfare, Health, and Cultural Affaires. The Hague, Government Publishing Office, 1983

Freud A, Burlingham DT: War and children. New York, Medical War Books, 1943

Glass AJ: Psychological aspects of disaster. Journal of the American Medical Association 171:222, 1959

Gur D, Good WF, Tokuhata GK, et al: Radiation-dose assignment to individuals residing near Three Mile Island Nuclear Station. Proceedings of the Pennsylvania Academy of Science 57:99–102, 1983

Hall E, Perlmutter M, Lamb ME: Child Psychology Today. New York, Random House, 1982

Howard SJ, Gordon NS: Final progress report: mental health investigation in a major disaster. Van Nuys, Calif, San Fernando Valley Child Guidance Clinic (NIMH Small Resource Grant MH 21649-01), 1972

Ingle DJ, Fisher GT: Effects of adrenalectomy during gestation on size of adrenals in newborn rats. Proc Soc Exp Biol Med 39:149–150, 1938

Jones JM, Lloyd CW, Wyatt TC: A study of the interrelationships of maternal and fetal adrenal glands of rats. Endocrinology 53:182–191, 1953

Josimovich JB, Hadman AJ, Deane HW: A histophysiological study of the developing adrenal cortex of the rat during fetal and early postnatal stages. Endocrinology 54:627–639, 1954

Kristal L: Bruxism: An anxiety response to environmental stress, in Stress and Anxiety, vol. 5. Edited by Spielberger CD, Sarason IG, Milgram NA. New York, Hemisphere/McGraw-Hill, 1978

Laube J, Murphy SA: Perspectives on Disaster Recovery. Norwalk, Conn, Appleton-Century-Crofts, 1985

McWhirter L, Trew K: Children in Northern Ireland: a lost generation? in The Child in His Family: Tomorrow's Parents. Edited by Anthony EJ, Chiland C. New York, John Wiley & Sons, 1982

Newman CJ: Children of disaster: clinical observations at Buffalo Creek. Am J Psychiatry 133(3):306–312, 1976

Rofe Y, Lewin I: Daydreams in a war environment. Journal of Mental Imagery 4:59–75, 1980

Sontag LW: Implications of fetal behavior and environment for adult personalities. Annals of the New York Academy of Sciences 134:782, 1966

Stern GM: The Buffalo Creek Disaster: The Story of the Survivors' Unprecedented Lawsuit. New York, Random House, 1976

Terr L: Psychic trauma in children: observations following the Chowchilla school-bus kidnapping. Am J Psychiatry 138:14–19, 1981

Thompson WR, Watson J, Charlesworth WR: The effects of prenatal maternal stress on offspring behavior in rats. Psychological Monographs: General and Applied 76:557, 1962

Tyhurst JS: Individual reactions to community disaster: the natural history of psychiatric phenomena. Am J Psychiatry 107:23–27, 1951

Upton AC: Health impact of the Three Mile Island accident: Health effect of ionizing radiation. Ann NY Acad Sci 365:63–75, 1981

Van der Ploeg HM: Identification of victims, with special reference to hostages, in Helping Victims of Violence. Edited by the Ministry of Welfare, Health, and Cultural Affaires, The Hague, Government Publishing Office, 1983

Ziv A, Kruglanski A, Shulman S: Children's psychological reactions to wartime stress. J Pers Soc Psychol 30:24–30, 1974

Chapter 5

Children Traumatized by Central American Warfare

William Arroyo, M.D.
Spencer Eth, M.D.

Chapter 5

Children Traumatized by Central American Warfare

Post-traumatic stress disorder (PTSD) (American Psychiatric Association 1980) is the most recent nomenclature for the collection of symptoms whose etiology is an external and overwhelming stress. The syndrome has been primarily studied in adults. These adults' lives have been significantly altered by the traumatic effects of various extreme stressors, including concentration camps (Hoppe 1968); civil and natural disasters (Erickson 1976; Green et al. 1983); rape (Burgess and Holmstrom 1974); and warfare (Kardiner and Spiegel 1947; Hendin et al. 1981). The Viet Nam War experience is probably the most common etiology of PTSD in the current American adult population. This particular population has been the primary focus of American PTSD research during the last decade (van der Kolk 1984).

Until recently the subject of psychic trauma in children has been only cursorily examined (Terr 1984). The significance of psychic trauma has now been clearly recognized in child abuse (Green 1983), kidnappings (Terr 1979), disasters (Newman 1976), the witnessing of parental homicide (Pynoos and Eth 1984), mutilating surgeries (Earle 1979), and war. The focus of this chapter is on childhood PTSD secondary to war-related trauma.

REVIEW OF LITERATURE

In general, the trauma that occurs during wartime is quite variable, consequently very difficult to assess, and even more burdensome to control for. Nevertheless, to study it is indispensable. Despite the monumental hindrances, the quality of the investigations of war-related traumas suffered by children steadily improved. The first authors to document these phenomena did so with reference to World War II. The results of these early studies varied from author to author.

One group of authors believed that children's reactions were very minimal in duration and intensity. For example, Freud and Burlingham (1942) concluded that war-traumatized children's reactions were primarily a function of the presence or absence of a parent or "familiar mother-substitute." Those children who experienced air raids did not seem particularly affected by them. In addition, they found that if a parent exhibited psychiatric symptoms secondary to the warfare, then the child often assumed a very similar symptom picture. Supporting their primary conclusions is Papanek (1942, 304). He deduced that when younger (age unspecified) children do not suffer physical injury from air raids, they ". . . measure the danger that threatens them chiefly by the reactions of those about them, especially of their trusted parents and teachers." Papanek treated some of these traumatized children, but neglected to describe his subject pool, methodology, and the specific stressors believed to have precipitated the psychiatric disturbances. Although anxiety is indicated as a prominent symptom in these children, other symptoms of PTSD are not clearly described.

Cyril Burt (1943, 325), who also studied British children from London and Liverpool, concurred with Anna Freud, "The nervous disturbances attributable to the war proved amazingly rare and amazingly slight." His main conclusion was that for physically uninjured children, "the mental shock of being bombed is in itself far less serious and persistent than the effect of having been in the company of an adult who has herself flown into a panic—possibly the child's own parent" (p. 324). Three-quarters of his cases under 16 years of age, who required evacuation because their homes were severely damaged, had psychiatric symptoms that resolved within a month. Without psychiatric follow-up and a more detailed description of symptoms, it is difficult to determine whether these children had adjustment disorders or PTSD. He also described a group of children having war "neuroses" resembling those reported in adult soldiers. This latter group may be closer to the PTSD symptom complex.

Another author who studied World War II British children was Carey-Trefzer (1949). She concluded that the most frequent symptom was an unspecified behavioral change followed by anxiety and fears. Bombardments, evacuations, and changes in family life were conjectured to be stressors more frequently resulting in psychiatric symptoms. Children of neurotic mothers showed reactions similar to their mother's reaction and more prolonged reactions. Nervous children were more prone to developing psychiatric symptoms, as Mercier (1943) and others found. Although PTSD cases were described by Carey-Trefzer, she concluded that a preexisting psychological factor was the etiology, not the actual trauma, in the majority of the cases.

Mercier (1943) and Mercier and Despert (1942), who studied the psychological effects of World War II on hundreds of French children, assumed the presence of several factors in the etiology of their subjects' symptoms. First, the children's reactions were a function of their personality. Second, their anxiety was manifested in terms of their "neurotic tendency" or prior emotional adjustment. And third, children were deemed to react to situations better than adults, though they often displayed their parents' attitudes. It was not evident that the authors believed that the symptom picture of delayed PTSD was the direct result of discrete war-related stressors.

Another group of European authors differed somewhat from the aforementioned authors. Dunsden (1941), for example, found that British children who remained under fire showed many more psychiatric disturbances than those who did not. Although his subjects and methods are not described, he portrayed both the acute and chronic types of PTSD.

Brander (1943), who studied Finnish children during the Russo-Finnish War of 1939–1940, documented PTSD in children as young as eight years old. He postulated a multifactorial etiology and recognized both types of PTSD in children who were exposed to warfare. The two most stressful factors were forced evacuation and air-raid alarms. He too found that "nervous" children became more so during wartime.

Observations of Spanish kindergarten children who lived in war zones were documented by Coromina (1943) during the late-1930s Spanish Civil War. Clearly noted were symptoms of anhedonia, isolation, depression, and a lessening of sociability in these youngsters. She concludes that the most potent stressors were evacuation and temporary placement in refugee camps.

The next group of war-related literature addresses young psychiatric casualties of the Southeast Asian, Middle Eastern, and South American Wars. In a study of psychiatric problems among adolescent Southeast Asian refugees, not one PTSD case was described (Williams and Westermeyer 1983). This is especially surprising since 5 of the 28 adolescents experienced the death of a parent. The duration of time between their entry to the United States and their examination is not indicated. Unless misdiagnosed, the more-prominent PTSD symptoms may have partially resolved prior to their becoming subjects.

Terrorist attacks on children in various parts of the world have precipatated PTSD in the young victims. Ayalon (1983) studied children and adolescents victimized by terrorists. These attacks are potentially more overwhelming than bombardments. Her study considers 10 different terrorist attacks on the Israeli civilian population between 1974 and 1980. Both acute and chronic PTSD are described. Two authors (Allodi 1980; Cohn et al. 1980) studied Chilean children with PTSD, who emigrated to Canada after their parents had been persecuted and then released from prison. The overwhelming majority were witnesses to the brutal arrest, torture, or execution of one or both parents. These types of stressors are infrequently described in the previously examined literature.

Ziv and Israeli (1973) studied children living in Kibbutzim. They concluded that bombardment did not separately contribute to the anxiety level of children. They conjecture that this may be due to a process of prolonged desensitization of the children to bombardments or that the instrument used to measure anxiety was not sufficiently sensitive. These results appear to contradict some of the World War II literature (Carey-Trefzer 1949, and others). Neither the frequency of the bombardments nor the proximity, which is probably the more-crucial variable, was mentioned in this study. This also may account for the negative findings. However, a study of the psychiatric sequelae of the 1969 Belfast Riots also downplays children's response to terrorism. The small number of children surveyed showed little early psychological reaction. "Indeed, as a rule, children appeared to enjoy the excitement, and parents described how they played in the barricades with toy guns" (Lyons 1971, 271). This activity may, in fact, be the children's attempt to master the severe stress they have experienced.

In summary, the diagnostic entity of what is now classified as PTSD, in children and adolescents who have been exposed to war-related trauma, has been documented in the medical literature throughout the last four decades. Most of the earlier literature was often anecdotal and the methodology was either poorly designed or not described at all. Some of the more-recent literature has also suffered from inadequate methodological procedures. Less than a handful of the studies have had control groups. These seemingly deficient methodologies are probably more a function of the evolution of warfare throughout the last century and the type of wars fought than a faulty design, per se. In addition, the precipitating stressors of PTSD seem to be of marked diversity, and multiple in the aforementioned studies. The actual stressor may, in fact, be a single one in most of the cases studied but because, among other reasons, several war-related stressors and their natural effects are difficult to disentangle and often present concomitantly and/or in rapid succession.

Despite the shortcomings of the various studies, two plausible conclusions can be made. First, war and extreme civil strife can adversely affect the local children and adolescents psychologically, and disrupt their normal development. And secondly, the more intimately (or personally) and catastrophically the youth are victimized, the greater is the risk of developing seriously disabling psychiatric symptoms.

CHILDREN FROM CENTRAL AMERICA

Civil strife has been endemic in several Central American countries. October 1979 marks the intensification of civil unrest in El Salvador. These Central American uprisings have precipitated a massive exodus of indigents fleeing for their personal safety. Hundreds of thousands of Salvadorans have escaped danger and resettled, in regions from Canada, in the north, to Argentina, in the south. The largest of the new Salvadoran refugee settlements consists of 400,000 members and is found in Los Angeles. The next-largest Central American group in Los Angeles is the Nicaraguan refugee cluster of 50,000 members. The majority of both groups are probably children.

Methods

Thirty Central American youngsters, 17 years of age or less, referred to the Los Angeles County–University of Southern California Division of Child/Adolescent Psychiatry comprise the subject pool of this investigation. All were exposed to warfare before entering the United States since January 1980. These children were referred by various local agencies including schools, the judicial system, pediatric hospitals, and other health agencies, whose personnel deemed that a psychiatric assessment was warranted. Each subject received a full psychiatric evaluation consisting of individual or family diagnostic interviews. In addition, a specialized interview protocol (Pynoos and Eth 1984) focusing on the exposure to warfare and associated violence was used with each subject.

Results and General Features of the Group

The presenting complaints among the subjects varied considerably. The range included suicidal behavior, multiple somatic complaints without organic etiology, various serious antisocial acts, insomnia, separation anxiety, defiance, and multiple school-related problems. The interval between arrival in the United States and the initial psychiatric contact varied from 3 weeks to 34 months. Twenty-eight of the subjects were from El Salvador; the remaining two were from Nicaragua.

Table 1 lists the *Diagnostic and Statistical Manual,* Third edition

Table 1. DSM-III Diagnoses Among 30 Central American Children

	Male	Female
Post-traumatic stress disorder	3	7
Adjustment disorders	4	5
Separation-anxiety disorder	2	0
Atypical somatoform disorder	2	0
Conversion disorder	0	1
Major depressive disorder	1	0
Conduct disorder	2	0
Dysthymic disorder	0	2
Schizophrenia, paranoid type	2	0
PCP intoxication	1	0
Parent–child problem	2	3

(*DSM-III*) diagnoses of the children, and their frequency. Several of the children had more than one diagnosis.

Of this group a total of six were hospitalized at the first psychiatric contact. The remainder were referred for outpatient treatment.

The children studied ranged in age from preschool to adolescence. Although certain generalizations across all ages have been made, phase-specific differences were also evident. Preschool children felt the most defenseless when faced with threat, and required the most assistance to recover. Because withdrawal is so common, very young children were mistakenly assumed to be unaffected by external events and were less commonly brought for psychiatric evaluation. But closer examination revealed characteristic symptoms of regression, including separation and stranger anxiety, frequent bed-wetting, irritability, and loss of acquired skills. Latency-age children presented primarily with school learning and conduct problems. Although it could have been anticipated that all immigrants would experience difficulties in a new school situation, these Central American children often fared far worse than other Hispanic cohorts. Their academic performance was impaired by the intrusion of traumatic memories and the peculiar stresses associated with parental separation and re-union. School-aged children displayed a diversity of behavioral changes, ranging from inhibition to aggression. They also reported a variety of somatic complaints, and would often be referred by a pediatrician when no organic basis was found for their psychosomatic symptoms. Adolescents were distinctively plagued by their tendency to engage in serious acting-out behavior. As a group, they exhibited the most aggression, directed toward other youth, new family members, and themselves (in the form of suicidal acts and drug abuse). Delinquency and out-of-wedlock pregnancy often brought them into contact with public agencies. A few adolescents were psychotic, and their typically paranoid delusions incorporated elements of their real-life experiences with the civil warfare.

Poverty was a major problem for the majority of these families prior to the outbreak of war. In several instances the children begged in the streets for food. Most had siblings who had died from infectious diseases secondary to the unavailability of medical care. In El Salvador, a quarter of all children die before the age of five.

Several of the children had already been victims or witnesses of major domestic violence. In two families, the father had been physically abusive of the mother. Two sisters, at ages 8 and 10, were repeatedly sexually assaulted by their father.

Prior to the war one father and one child were treated for generalized anxiety disorder, and two teenagers were treated for PTSD.

The parents of half of the children and adolescents emigrated to the United States as early as several years before their offspring. These children were left with other family members or designated guardians.

Five single mothers, who emigrated several years before their children, remarried and bore at least one child prior to the arrival in the United States of the subjects.

Case Descriptions

The following two case studies of children with PTSD will illustrate the series of severe stressors that these children experienced and in some instances, barely survived.

Case #1. Esperanza is an attractive 17-year-old Salvadoran, who entered the United States four months prior to her initial psychiatric contact. She was referred by a free clinic where she was primarily examined for a one-year history of a dull, left-sided headache associated with a strange sensation in her left eye. Her pain was occasionally precipitated by anger, was unresponsive to over-the-counter analgesics, and resolved spontaneously. In addition, she complained of various psychological symptoms.

Esperanza was born out-of-wedlock; her father is unknown. She was raised by her mother and a "good" stepfather, who divorced her mother when she was five. There were many days when she and her two half brothers were without food. At other times the mother was negligent.

At age seven she and her half siblings were left with her maternal aunt under the pretext the mother was going on an errand. The mother in fact emigrated to the United States, and Esperanza remained with her aunt, whom she came to prefer and whom she guiltily refers to as "mother."

At the age of 14 she joined a politically active pro-government organization, in which she received formal training in the use of firearms. She did not engage in violence. After quitting 1 year later, she joined an antigovernment organization, with the encouragement of her cousins, who were members. Two of these cousins subsequently became *desaparecidos* (missing persons). At the age of 15, one of her official duties was to lead, on a weekly basis, a group of mothers of *desaparecidos* to the local morgue. There the weeping mothers ambivalently hoped to identify one of the (often-mutilated, dismembered, or burned) corpses as that of a son or daughter.

Becoming concerned about Esperanza's involvement in political activity, the mother sent for her. After an embittered and protested two-week stay in the United States, 15-year-old Esperanza returned to El Salvador.

Two months later she was beaten for her verbal protests during the military's interrogation of her 18-year-old male cousin. She was incarcerated for two days and raped by the jail security. She was apparently hit on the head prior to being raped and could not recall many details of the rape. In fact, she was not certain that she had been raped until it was confirmed by a self-examination of her genital area along with a verbal confirmation by another prisoner.

She and her cousin fled to Mexico to seek refuge after receiving a series of threats by government officials. In Mexico they were granted political asylum and provided with shelter and part-time employment for one and one-half years. During her stay she frequently became depressed, made several suicide gestures, developed headaches, and exhibited various other signs of PTSD.

Prior to the termination of the provision of quarters in Mexico, Esperanza and her cousin accepted her mother's invitation to join her while their applications for political asylum in the United States and Canada were processed. Her relationship with her natural mother resumed its stormy and antagonistic course. Esperanza and her mother frequently argued. At one point, the mother secretly and unsuccessfully instructed her daughter's immigration attorney to withdraw the political-asylum application.

Both the Canadian and American Immigration Departments denied Esperanza political asylum. She was ordered to leave the United States within three weeks, after which date, if apprehended, she would be involuntarily repatriated. She remained in Los Angeles, often terrified by the thought of being deported and killed by the military upon arrival to El Salvador. She compared her current fright to that when she was pursued in El Salvador after her release from prison.

Her initial mental status examination revealed an appropriately groomed and dressed, dark-skinned, attractive teenager who appeared her stated age. Her mental status seemed unremarkable except for a depressed mood.

The fact that she had not made a suicide attempt nor considered suicide during the last six months was evidence that she had improved considerably since being assaulted two years previously, she claimed. It was actually her general state which betrayed the initial picture of an attractive, minimally depressed, teenage girl. In Mexico, her social life had been limited to her employment as a part-time domestic. After being victimized and emigrating to Mexico, she had lost her interest in socializing and dating, which contrasted greatly with her social life in El Salvador. She described her various experiences, which were overwhelming and horrifying to most people, with a strikingly constricted affect. Her sleep was repeatedly disrupted by nightmares during the last year but less so now (3–4/week) than initially. The content of most of her nightmares was war-related. The most frequently repeated dream was one in which she is beaten by soldiers who subsequently restrain her with belts. She did not recall any rape-related dreams. Although her memory and concentration had become impaired after the assaults, they were less so than initially. She often avoided discussing the assaults. Her cousin described two dissociative-like states during which she frightfully stared and screamed for approximately two minutes. She was described as being completely indistractible during these states.

Her initial *DSM-III* diagnosis is post-traumatic stress disorder, chronic type, and dysthymic disorder.

Case #2. Pedro, a newly arrived, five-year-old Salvadoran boy, was referred for multiple symptoms by a pediatrician.

Father and mother emigrated separately to the United States when Pedro was one and two years old, respectively. He and his two older sisters remained under the care of their maternal aunt and maternal grandfather, who was a military officer, in a rural town.

The children were frequent witnesses to aerial bombings of nearby residences, which went up in flames, producing immense clouds of smoke. These incidents prompted the children to seek refuge underneath the bed, where Pedro often wept inconsolably for his mother. At other times, the sudden sounds of bombings precipitated periods of severe tremulousness in Pedro. Periodically, raids were also conducted at nearby residences, which resulted in the local streets being openly riddled with corpses. The sight of automobiles, which were only driven by military officers, often precipitated intense fear in Pedro.

His parents finally sent for Pedro, five, and his sisters, six and seven, after learning of the children's worsening condition.

The children's reunion with their parents was delayed upon their entry into the United States. The children, along with an adult female "coyote" (alien smuggler), were apprehended by U.S. immigration officers in Tucson. The children were then relocated to Phoenix, where they were housed separately for three weeks from the coyote, who claimed to be their mother.

In Phoenix they resided in a one-room structure with a female immigration officer who interacted minimally with the children. They were prohibited from going outside. Each child was fed one meal per day consisting of a sandwich and a glass of juice.

Pedro's parents, who were living in Los Angeles, were finally invited to identify their children in Phoenix. Because of inadequate financial resources, the father traveled alone in an attempt to regain his children. To the father's dismay, only the older daughter recognized him. This observation by the immigration officials, coupled with the coyote's claim to be the children's mother, led to the father's returning home alone. This resulted in more-frequent crying spells in the children, and a nearly complete loss of hope of ever reuniting with their parents.

Two weeks later an arrangement was made to transfer the children to Los Angeles, where their mother would attempt to reclaim them. The children were placed behind a glass partition through which they could view their mother. When the mother appeared, the three children burst into tears and were allowed to join her for a few minutes. The officials then forcibly separated the clinging children while the mother completed the proper immigration documents. This, of course, precipitated much more screaming and terror in the children.

The family now lives in an apartment in a poverty-stricken neighborhood. The mother reports that Pedro hears gunshots at least weekly around the apartment complex and recently saw two nearby apartments engulfed in flames; each of these events has precipitated severe panic attacks.

In addition to being terrified by the sound of gunshots, Pedro consistently exhibits precipitous startle reactions at the sight and/or sound of airplanes, smoke and fire, and certain vans, which he fears might actually belong to military officers. Irritability, crying episodes, tremulousness, and anorexia for up to 24 hours after each startle reaction are noted. He becomes intensely fearful when the whereabouts of his sisters are unknown and when a parent is not in sight. Headaches also frequently follow the startle reactions. When frightened, he is noted to become "very pale" and more quiet than usual. While asleep he becomes very restless and occasionally cries. He generally cannot recall his "scary" nightmares but was able to relate the following one. He had awakened one evening to the sounds and sight of his home being bombed and suddenly discovered that he was alone.

At the initial visit, Pedro appeared with his parents and two older sisters. He sat lodged between his mother and father. Pedro was remarkably reluctant to engage in any verbal exchange and to separate from his parents. With parental prompting he responded to questions in a barely audible voice and in two- and three-word sentences. He repeatedly played with the available toy soldiers, positioning the military forces on one side and the guerillas on the other and then knocking them down with one quick handstroke stating that they all died because they were all bad.

His understanding of the situation in his homeland was limited to fear and to soldiers and guerillas killing one another for unknown reasons. He also knew that his parents had been waiting for him in a distant place.

His initial diagnoses were post-traumatic stress disorder and separation-anxiety disorder.

DISCUSSION

Post-traumatic stress disorder in both cases is assumed to be a direct result of the discrete traumatic events that each child experienced. In the first case description, both the violent beating and the rape are the traumatic events presumably responsible for the manifestation of PTSD. In the second, the aerial bombardments appear to be most directly associated with the child's symptoms. But, in fact, in addition to the overwhelming stressors of inflicted injury, rape, and bombings, this study group of children and adolescents has undergone a series of agonizing stressors, which modifies the psychiatric symptom complex, its duration, and, ultimately, its resolution.

Privation affected most of these children and adolescents early in life in Central America. The lack of shelter, the low protein–caloric intake, and the paucity of medical services have significantly contributed to the elevated child-mortality rate. This privation has probably adversely affected their growth, development, central nervous system maturation, and attachment behavior, all of which predispose to psychopathology.

It is difficult to understand the rationale of those mothers who emigrated early and who were perceived by their children as abandoning them. Perhaps the stress of extreme poverty, the consequent impairment of family relationships (Parmelee et al. 1983), and the constant danger from civil war figured in the mother's decision to extrude these children in order to protect herself and more-cherished family members.

The overwhelming majority of children who witnessed the war-related violence were threatened with death if they, as one child stated, "brought any attention," displayed any emotion, or identified the corpses which littered the streets. These children remained in a painful state of forced silence (Lister 1982). This death threat further psychologially compromised a substantial number of these already-traumatized youngsters. In at least two cases this intense fear was evident for some time after arrival in the United States.

The majority of subjects had great difficulty in providing clear accounts of their many psychological insults. Each episode tended to blend into a montage of frightening memories of overwhelming anxiety and helplessness. Their sequencing of the traumatic events was frequently inaccurate. This finding was more prominent in the younger children, as with Terr's kidnap victims (1983). The multiple traumas seem to have caused a long-term impairment in remote memory. As their poor school performance implies, other cognitive functions were affected as well. The difficulty of collecting historical information was compounded by the absence of the caretaker who was responsible for the child during the stressful periods, who generally remained in Central America.

Several developmental lines were disrupted by the civil strife. Psychosocial and moral development of some of these youngsters were altered. Many of the children were restricted to indoors. The parents of these house-bound children feared for their children's safety on the streets, and in some cases the children themselves become highly sensitized to the startling sounds of bombs and to the terrorizing sights of fire, as in the second case described. Social activities were limited because school activities were repeatedly disrupted and therefore parents preferred their children to be at home. The adolescents diminished their outdoor activities to avoid being forcibly enlisted with one of the factions. In some of the rural communities youngsters below the age of 14 were being trained and armed for combat. Many of these youngsters continued to exhibit several incapacitating avoidant behaviors after arrival in the United States.

The sanctioned display and encouragement of violent aggression by adult role models, who repeatedly terrorized, tortured, murdered, and destroyed, presents an overpowering challenge to the children's developing efforts at impulse control. The increased incidence of adolescent antisocial behavior during war is well documented (Carey-Trefzer 1949; Mercier and Despert 1942). After being arrested in the United States for a minor offense, one newly arrived male teenager retorted that his crime was nothing in comparison to the violent crimes adults commit in his former homeland. Grinberg and Grinberg (1984, 33) have commented that under conditions of forced immigration the process of integration is usually more painful: "There is more bitterness; hate directed against his own country is greater and, absurd as it may appear, this is projected into the receiving country."

Like Esperanza, the children whose parents emigrated early were often left behind without any preparation. Others were left in the care of irresponsible and abusive guardians. As in the second case study, some of the separations were so prolonged or so early in the child's life that, upon reunion with the natural parent(s), the child could no longer recognize the parent. In others the infant bonded to the new guardian. In three cases the child rejoiced in anticipation of reuniting with his or her mother in the United States, only to discover a new father and new half siblings. The impact of unexpected and unwelcomed family members seriously jeopardized the young and fearful immigrant's adjustment to his or her new home and surroundings.

Another group of children exists whose additional features must be considered separately. These are those who directly participated in combat; two members of this pool were combatants before the age of 16. They became both terrified and remorseful of the memories of their participation in the torture and massacres of fellow citizens and neighbors. As with the Viet Nam veteran, "participation in and witnessing abusive violence are two additional measures of war stress found to be important in assessing the effects of the war experience" (Laufer et al. 1984, 64). Like Gault's (1971) subjects, the two teenagers frequently addressed the atrocities they witnessed; but, both reluctantly recounted their own participation. Haley (1974) discusses the necessary sensitivity with which one must approach these former combatants.

Guerrilla warfare differs from the conventional type of warfare in that it is usually even more stressful (Laufer et al. 1984). In a guerrilla campaign it can be extremely difficult for both civilians and combatants to distinguish between the opposing forces.

Like the young Viet Nam veteran, the idealistic adolescent Salvadoran soldier has "experienced traumatic disillusionment with the military establishment" (Jackson 1982, 229) and is unable to integrate the combat stress. This results in what Jackson calls a prolonged arrest in a phase of moral nihilism interfering with superego consolidation. Later encounters with Los Angeles youth gangs, the illicit drug trade, and deportation raids serve to confirm the child's perception of the apparent immorality of the adult world.

Immigration for most of the children and all of the adolescents proved to be an additional source of stress. This process increased their dependence on their parents or other adults. For many adolescents it was a regressive step into childhood, as they mobilized their efforts to accomplish a cultural transition along with other necessary developmental tasks.

The actual entry into the United States was, at the very least, moderately anxiety provoking. In other cases, as for Pedro, it consisted of a sequence of severe stressors. For those children unaccompanied by their parents, the threat of not finding a parent became acute when they crossed the Mexico–United States border in the custody of a coyote. Parents routinely depleted their savings in order to smuggle their children to the United States. Often when their children arrive in Los Angeles the parents are unable to provide them with the basic necessities of life.

The resettlement phase along with the uprooting and actual emigration were so stressful as to precipitate different types of adjustment reactions in all age groups. In addition to expending energy on the arduous task of learning a new language, adopting new customs, surviving gang-riddled neighborhoods, the adolescents ruminated incessantly about the threat of deportation. Unlike the other recent waves of political refugees entering the United States, this group is neither welcomed nor provided with concrete services such as food, shelter, and routine medical care. As undocumented aliens, Central American immigrants are not entitled to the standard benefits of aid to families with dependent children, food stamps, or medicaid (medi-Cal). However, the children are eligible to enroll in public school and by state law can receive mental health care (which permitted this study). Less than 1 percent of all political-asylum applications by Salvadorans during 1980 to 1983 have been granted by the U.S. Immigration and Naturalization Service.

CONCLUSION

These Central American refugee youngsters have been targets of various assaults, with each assault varying in its developmental point of entry, its intensity, its duration, and its psychopathological result. Unfortunately, the chronically malnourished and deprived young child is compromised early. As with the child who's immunologically suppressed and vulnerable to virulent infectious agents, the war-ravaged child who has experienced traumatic stress is gravely predisposed to further opportunistic insults in the form of separations, a forced uprooting, and a tumultuous resettlement. However, having identified their special circumstances, the war-traumatized child's prognosis becomes more favorable with further study and timely interventions. As a growing segment of our society, it is essential that some preparation be made to adequately meet the needs of this special population.

REFERENCES

Allodi F: The psychiatric effects in children and families of victims of political persecution and torture. Danish Medical Bulletin 27:229–232, 1980

American Psychiatric Association: Diagnostic and Statistical Manual of Mental Disorders, 3rd ed. Washington, DC, American Psychiatric Association, 1980

Ayalon O: Coping with terrorism, in Stress in Israel. Edited by Breznitz S. New York, Van Nostrand Reinhold Co, 1983

Brander T: Psychiatric observations among Finnish children during the Russo–Finnish War of 1939–1940. The Nervous Child 2:313–319, 1943

Burgess A, Holmstrom L: Rape: Victims of Crisis. Bowie, Md, Robert J. Brady Co, 1974

Burt C: War neuroses in British children. Nervous Child 2:324–337, 1943

Carey-Trefzer C: The results of a clinical study of war-damaged children who attended the child guidance clinic, the Hospital for Sick Children, Great Ormand Street, London. The Journal of Mental Science 95:535–559, 1949

Cohn J, Kirsten IMH, Koch L, et al: Children and torture. Danish Medical Bulletin 27:238-239, 1980

Coromina J: Repercussions of the war on children as observed during the Spanish Civil War. The Nervous Child 2:324–337, 1943

Dunsdon MI: A psychologist's contribution to air-raid problems. Ment Health 2:37–41, 1941

Earle E: The psychological effects of mutilating surgery in children and adolescents. Psychoanal Study Child 34:527–546, 1979

Erikson K: Everything in Its Path—Destruction of Community in the Buffalo Creek Flood. New York, Simon and Shuster, 1976

Freud A, Burlingham D (1942): Report 12, in The Writings of Anna Freud, vol. 3. New York, International Universities Press, 1973

Gault WB: Some remarks on slaughter. Am J Psychiatry 128:4:82–85, 1971

Green A: Dimension of psychological trauma in abused children. J Am Acad Child Psychiatry 22:231–237, 1983

Green BL, Grace MC, Lindy JD, et al: Levels of functional impairment following a civilian disaster: the Beverly Hills Supper Club fire. J Consult Clin Psychol 51:573–580, 1983

Grinberg L, Grinberg R: A psychoanalytic study of migration: its normal and pathological aspects. J Am Psychoanal Assoc 32:13–38, 1984

Haley SA: When the patient reports atrocities. Arch Gen Psychiatry 30:191–196, 1974

Hendin H, Haas AP, Singer P, et al: Meanings of combat and the development of post-traumatic stress disorder. Am J Psychiatry 138:1490–1493, 1981

Hoppe KD: Psychotherapy with concentration-camp survivors, in Massive Psychic Trauma. Edited by Kristal H. New York, International Universities Press, 1968

Husain SA, Vandiver T: Suicide in Children and Adolescents. New York, Spectrum Publications, 1984

Jackson HC: Moral nihilism: Developmental arrest as a sequel to combat stress, in Adolescent Psychiatry, vol 10. Edited by Feinstein SC, Looney JG, Schwartzberg AZ, et al. Chicago, University of Chicago Press, 1982

Kardiner A, Spiegel H: War Stress and Neurotic Illness. New York, Hoeber, 1947

Laufer RS: Post-traumatic stress disorder (PTSD) reconsidered: PTSD among Viet Nam veterans, in Post Traumatic Stress Disorder: Psychological and Biological Sequelae. Edited by van der Kolk BA. Washington, DC, American Psychiatric Press, 1984

Lister ED: Forced silence: a neglected dimension of trauma. Am J Psychiatry 139:872–875, 1982

Lyons HA: Psychiatric sequelae of the Belfast riots. Br J Psychiatry 118:265–273, 1971

Mercier MH: The suffering of French children. The Nervous Child 2:308–312, 1943

Mercier MH, Despert JL: Psychological effects of the war on French children. Psychosom Med 5:266–272, 1942

Newman CJ: Children of disaster: clinical observations at Buffalo Creek. Am J Psychiatry 133:306–312, 1976

Papanek E: My experiences with fugitive children in Europe. Nervous Child 2:301–307, 1942

Parmelee A, Beckwith L, Cohen S, et al: Social influences on infants at medical risk for behavioral difficulties, in Frontiers of Infant Psychiatry, 1st ed. Edited by Call JD, Galenson E, Tyson RL. New York, Basic Books, 1983

Pynoos R, Eth S: Child as witness to homicide. J Soc Issues 40:87–108, 1984

Pynoos R, Eth S: Witness to violence: the child interview. J Am Acad Child Psychiatry (in press)

Terr LC: Children of Chowchilla: a study of psychic trauma. Psychoanal Study Child 34:547–623, 1979

Terr LC: Time sense following psychic trauma. Am J Orthopsychiatry 53:244–261, 1983

Terr LC: Children at acute risk: psychic trauma, in Psychiatry Update, vol. 3. Edited by Grinspoon L. Washington, DC, American Psychiatric Press, 1984, pp 104–120

van der Kolk BA: Post-Traumatic Stress Disorder: Psychological and Biological Sequelae. Washington, DC, American Psychiatric Press, 1984

Williams CL, Westermeyer J: Psychiatric problems among adolescent Southeast Asian refugees: a descriptive study. J Nerv Ment Dis 171:79–85, 1983

Ziv A, Israeli R: Effects of bombardment on the manifest anxiety level of children living in Kibbutzim. J Consult Clin Psychol 40:287–291, 1973

Ziv A, Kruglanski A, Shulman S: Children's psychological reactions to wartime stress. J Pers Soc Psychol 30:24–30, 1974

Chapter 6

Post-Traumatic Stress Disorder in Children with Cancer

Yehuda Nir, M.D.

Chapter 6

Post-Traumatic Stress Disorder in Children with Cancer

During the last decade medical advances in pediatric oncology have significantly increased the survival rate of children with cancer. Such progress, while welcomed, has serious consequences for the child. A cure or extended life span is a result of prolonged and aggressive treatment, chemotherapy, radiotherapy, and surgery, either separately or in combination for periods of up to five years. On a daily basis the treatment may include painful venipunctures, spinal taps, and bone marrow aspirations. Chemotherapy and radiation cause loss of appetite, nausea, vomiting, painful mucosal ulcerations, weakness (necessitating prolonged bed rest), and loss of hair. These are grave consequences of the therapy that confront the child.

The diagnosis of cancer plunges a child into this new medical reality, creating a series of overwhelming problems for young patients and their families. The issues are both physical and emotional in nature. Although initially distinct, in the course of the child's illness, the physical and emotional components tend to interdigitate, often becoming almost indistinguishable from one another.

In view of these complexities, psychological input and understanding of all the elements that come into contact with the sick child are essential, not only to assure optimal medical intervention, but to support the emotional well-being of the child. Koocher and O'Malley's (1981) study has shown that the child who is cured from cancer, while physically well, runs the risk of remaining emotionally handicapped.

In our attempt to effectively assist the child with cancer we began to explore the particular nature of psychological reactions that accompany this illness, as well as ways to diagnose the emotional components of the disease. In order to arrive at a reliable assessment we have applied the diagnostic criteria of the third edition of the *Diagnostic and Statistical Manual of Mental Disorders* (*DSM-III*, American Psychiatric Association 1980). Our assessment, which consists of both clinical interviews and psychological testing, leads to a conclusion that the primary psychopathology encountered in the majority of child and adolescent patients with cancer falls into the diagnostic criteria of the post-traumatic stress disorder (PTSD). In our evaluation procedures we have been struck by the extent to which so many of our patients fulfill all the diagnostic criteria of PTSD, with the length of illness being an important variable in determining status in either the acute, chronic, or delayed categories.

DIAGNOSTIC CRITERIA IN POST-TRAUMATIC STRESS DISORDER AND THEIR CLINICAL SIGNIFICANCE IN CHILDHOOD CANCER

Stress

Stress, in reaction to the diagnosis and treatment of cancer, is ubiquitous. It is intensified, in the case of childhood cancer, by the fact that it is so totally unexpected and that its life-threatening aspects upset the natural order—children die before their parents. Though stress seems unavoidable, the extent of its impact seems to depend on several variables: the type of cancer diagnosed; whether the child is in a high-, medium-, or low-risk group; the location of the tumor; the age of the patient; the constellation of the family; whether another member of the family has had cancer; and whether a member of the family has died of cancer in the recent past.

The child's ability to cope with the stress of cancer will play an important role in the way he or she deals with the illness itself and with the treatment, which can be an overwhelming experience. Feelings of helplessness and vulnerability dominate this stage, often leading to regressive behavior in the very young, the latency, and the adolescent patient. The regressive behavior is age-specific and usually reflects the developmental stage of the sick child. Withdrawal and active refusal to participate in the treatment are seen almost immediately at the onset of the disease in both the very young and latency children. As these types of behavior interfere with the medical management of a life-threatening illness, there seems to be no time available to help the child to overcome the maladaptive style of coping with trauma. Instead, the resistance to treatment is circumvented by the use of general anesthesia, hypnotic relaxation techniques, or insertion of a Broviac catheter, which eliminates the need for intravenous needles. All these interventions, while medically justified, intensify the feelings of passivity and helplessness, lowering the threshold for additional stress.

In adolescence, the feelings of helplessness may become sexualized.

A 17-year-old female patient with acute lymphocytic leukemia (ALL) reported the following dream after having refused chemotherapy: "Two doctors are forcefully holding me down while the third one is shoving pills down her throat." Another adolescent girl coped with loss of control by becoming sexually active. This resulted in a pregnancy between two courses of chemotherapy. "I don't have time to wait," was her explanation. Regression can also take form of acute separation anxiety; we have observed young children, whose parents cannot stay overnight in the hospital, falling asleep with telephone receivers in their laps after having talked to their parents, as if to maintain contact with what has become elusive.

Since the intensity and nature of the stressor color the clinical course of the disease, it should become an important consideration in any type of psychosocial intervention. Some stressors are easily identifiable and can be dealt with immediately, at the time of diagnosis. For example, those related to the family constellation. Specifically, we have observed that divorced or separated parents may have a detrimental effect on the patient's treatment, particularly when conflicts about decision making (often centering around the signing of informed-consent forms) exist. Preventing parental discord, which can compromise a child's well-being and the physician's ability to treat the patient effectively, is essential. Addressing this issue at the time of diagnosis can assure a conjoint effort in the best interest of the child.

More generally, in our work in childhood cancer we have learned to view the parental coping style as a potential stressor—if it is maladaptive. By contrast, it serves to neutralize stress—if the coping style is adaptive. However, it is of critical importance that the parental coping style be congruent with that of the child if it is to serve to augment the child's adaptive defense mechanisms.

As observed by Tan et al. (1983), families that seem best equipped to cope are those who can develop a therapeutic alliance with the pediatric oncologist to work conjointly through the vicissitudes of the illness. This requires a high degree of ego maturity and sophistication from parents and pediatrician alike. Their alliance serves to buffer and protect the child from much of the pain and stress of the daily treatment regimen.

Another subgroup of parents who seem successful in reducing stress are those with strong religious beliefs. It seems as if unwavering acceptance and faith offer the child stability, a sense of predictability, that can serve to soften the impact of the harsh realities of the illness and its management.

By contrast, parents who raise the level of stress display a variety of maladaptive defenses. We have labeled one high-stress parental style *aggressive pursuers*. These parents "shop" for what they consider to be the best possible treatment, often in total disregard of the child's needs and wishes (and even physical condition). They find the possibility of the child's death unacceptable and pursue treatment against all odds. Striking evidence of this style of coping became clear to us in our recent randomized study (Tan et al. 1983) of 26 parents who elected to have their children receive experimental phase I drugs. Post-treatment interviews revealed that none of the parents were aware of the fact that the informed-consent form, signed at the time of treatment, specifically stressed that no therapeutic response can be expected from the drug. The need to take action seemed the paramount concern. The aggressive pursuer intensifies the traumatic experience of the child as their frenetic activity heightens the child's feeling of vulnerability and undermines his/her trust in the medical establishment.

Other parents who intensify the stress of childhood cancer are those who employ intellectual, obsessive–compulsive defense mechanisms as a way of contending with the situation. Frequently professionals, they try to obtain as much information as possible about the child's illness, checking and rechecking the oncologist's decisions and actions. Their behavior interferes with the forging of a therapeutic alliance, and often stimulates defensive medicine. Anticipation and fear of parental reaction intrudes on countless therapeutic decisions. Children of parents who use this style of coping are in a particular predicament, namely, on the one hand, they are reassured by the total attention of their parents, which extends into the realm of medical treatment; on the other, there is a thinly veiled message that the doctors cannot be trusted. This ambiguity intensifies the anxiety level in the child.

Another problematic coping style is most apparent among fathers of adolescent male patients. It is invariably influenced by their identification with their sons. A thinly veiled attempt to neutralize overwhelming anxiety, it often surfaces as a macho-type attitude. For example, following an above-the-knee amputation, the father of a 12-year-old boy with osteosarcoma wrote on the bandaged stump "bitten off by a shark" and insisted that the boy join him on a fishing trip two days after surgery. Parental coping style may intrude on the child's ability to handle effectively the stress of having cancer if it interferes with what Lazarus (1977) described as a change of perception, from experiencing the stressor as a threat, to seeing it as a challenge to one's sense of mastery. If this transition does not take place, the patient might respond with a passive submission to both disease and procedures and assume a victim–martyr identity. Here again, the adolescent patient seems most vulnerable. The overanxious or controlling parent might use the illness as a way of reestablishing control over the child, who had begun to assume an age-appropriate independence prior to the onset of illness. As one 16-year-old stated: "I sometimes don't know who is sick, me or my mother."

Intrusive Recollections, Repetitious Dreams, Nightmares

The second diagnostic criterion of PTSD deals with intrusive recollections, the presence of repetitious dreams, and nightmares. Our observations, as well those of others, consistently indicate the presence of such phenomena in children with cancer. Koocher and O'Malley (1981) addressed this problem succinctly, having coined the term the Damocles Syndrome—which describes the omnipresent fear of relapse that haunts the child—no matter how many years have passed since the treatment that produced cure. Child and family live with the potential for continuous evocation of retraumatization. One adolescent cured from Hodgkin's disease experienced fears and nightmares whenever she felt aches in her legs, since she thought of such aches as the first signs of her original cancer. In another family, a child who had suffered from an abdominal mass became periodically hysterical when any of her siblings complained of stomachaches. In this same family, any somatic distress resulted in immediate "emergency" medical consultation. Nausea may often intrude on a child's life as a recurrent memory of reaction to past chemotherapy. Sometimes a psychosomatic symptom may be the trigger for recollection of a traumatic experience and be accompanied by an anxiety attack. Such is the vulnerability to the intrusive somatic stimuli that some patients express a desire to have a drastic but definite procedure, rather than a less-invasive but ambiguous intervention. The following case will explain this point. A 19-year-old male with osteosarcoma of his right knee had, following the course of chemotherapy, his knee replaced with a mechanically functional implant. The complicated procedure and subsequent recovery were uneventful and the patient was able to walk without support. Nevertheless, he requested, six months later, to have his right leg amputated, as he found the idea of having a metal implant in his leg intolerable. He became obsessed with fears of falling down, fracturing his leg, osteomyelitis, total loss of the leg, and eventual death as a result of all the complications. According to his surgeon, there was no medical justification for his concerns. The patient anticipated that the finality and predictability of an amputation will relieve him of his fears.

Such painful intrusions are the long-term legacy of childhood cancer, although the stimulus for an intrusive recollection may seem minor to the outside observer. In response to these stimuli, repression becomes easily reversable. We have observed a very specific defense strategy aimed at suppressing the omnipresent intrusive reminders of the life-threatening condition. Cathexis is shifted from the illness to treatment. Chemotherapy, injections, bone-marrow aspirations become the central preoccupation of children and parents. The "battleground" where treatment takes place serves as a diversion from the threat of cancer. A 12-year-old patient who has had ALL since age 3 said, "I never saw any signs of my illness, all I was worried about was losing my hair again" (S. La Farge, personal communication). Counterphobic behavior is a common defense mechanism in these children. It is seen primarily in amputees and children with hematological disorders like the Evan syndrome, where uncontrollable bleeding can be life threatening. We have seen children with bleeding disorders learning karate or other martial arts, while many amputees drive regular cars with one leg or dive or jump on one leg (Nir 1979).

It is important for the psychiatrist involved in the treatment of the child with cancer to know the many permanent physical sequelae of cancer, since these play a significant role in leaving the child more susceptible to retraumatization. Nerve damage due to the drug Vincristine and cognitive impairment due to cranial radiation in leukemia are common aftereffects. Mutilating surgery (for example amputations) and sterility due to either radiation, chemotherapy, or surgery are seen in large numbers of cured patients. These and other sequelae are unavoidable and lifelong reminders of the disease. The threat of a relapse, either the primary cancer or the appearance of a secondary malignancy (possibly as a result of radiation and chemotherapy treatment), places the child with cancer in a special, yet-unexplored subgroup of patients suffering PTSD. The lifelong potential for retraumatization is unique for this group as, unlike other repeatedly traumatized children (i.e., physically or psychologically abused children), there is no escape for the child with cancer. As cure in childhood cancer is a relatively new development, there aren't any truly longitudinal studies to assess the clinical manifestations of the PTSD that develops under these circumstances and with it, the long-term emotional impact of surviving cancer.

In fact, the inability to successfully repress the cancer experience, with its psychological and physical aftereffects, even in the event of complete cure, seems to be among the great challenges facing pediatric oncology. Attempting to meet this challenge, the Memorial Sloan Kettering Cancer Center in New York has added to its roster of task forces one on child psychiatry, in order to anticipate the needs of children cured from cancer in years to come.

Affect

In the area of affect the child with cancer also meets the diagnostic criteria for PTSD. Feelings of estrangement, primarily from the peer group and siblings, are most pronounced. Social isolation is exacerbated by loss of hair, prolonged absences from school, and peer group avoidance of the sick child. Prejudices as to the contagion of cancer and projective identification with the patient add to the isolation experience. Isolation, when prolonged, will intensify the child's dependence on the parents at the expense of peer contact. In an adolescent it might intrude on age-specific developmental tasks, namely, the renegotiation of separation and individuation. The conflict centers around dependency, with its concomitant increased security in the threatening illness, versus independence and pursuit of age-appropriate tasks and relationships. If the course of the illness becomes protracted, the dependence may lead to a lifelong disability in interpersonal relation. A 22-year-old patient, dying of secondary cancer following treatment for Hodgkin's disease at 16, stated that she regretted that she went, at her parents' insistence, to college at 18. "I should have gotten married and had a child, to capture at least a part of my short life." Physical handicaps like amputations, fatigue due to chemotherapy, or low blood counts prevent a youngster with cancer from participating in sports, an important medium for socializing, adding to the feeling of isolation. An additional factor that increases estrangement is academic failure due to cancer. It may be psychogenic (i.e., lack of interest as a reflection of a depressive affective component); physiologic, due to cranial radiation (Tamaroff et al. 1982); or the result of prolonged absences from school. Loneliness and sadness are often the emotional aftermath of what is often a frightening experience as well. The convergence of these factors can have a highly disruptive impact on the child's functioning.

Depression

The more pathological symptoms of PTSD (depression, hyperalertness, insomnia, and excessive irritability with aggressive or impulsive behavior) are often present, but are most likely to be observed in two types of patients; those with previous psychiatric history or psychiatric symptomology and those patients where a prolonged disease course (with many relapses over a period of years) has caused burnout, a feeling of battle fatigue with accompanying depression, insomnia, anorexia, and resignation.

The patient or family with psychopathology that antedates cancer presents a highly complicated situation. Frequently, they are perceived by the medical staff as uncooperative, undependable, and suspicious rather than as suffering from symptoms of a psychiatric disorder. To prevent this disruption in the patient–doctor relationship we have instituted a mandatory psychiatric examination for anyone with past psychiatric history. Short-term psychotherapy and/ or medication may follow the examination. Medical staff frequently comment on the relief they experience through this intervention— they are free to treat the child effectively rather than engage in nonproductive interactions with patients or families.

TREATMENT

The perception that a child with cancer is suffering from PTSD enabled us to gain a clearer perspective on the total psychiatric, clinical management of the child. It has also allowed us to deal with specified clinical manifestations within an understandable context. Having made these observations, what are the practical consequences?

Of all the symptoms that reflect PTSD, we have been most effective in dealing with stress-related aspects of the emotional reaction to childhood cancer. Early intervention with high-risk families has become a therapeutic imperative. They take the form of either direct psychiatric contact, social-work counseling, theme-centered groups, or assistance to medical staff in understanding the psychodynamics of behavior and interactions of both parents and child. The last type of intervention takes the form of weekly multidisciplinary psychosocial conferences. The high-risk patients are presented and intervention strategies deliberated.

We have been less effective in dealing with retraumatization and intrusive recollections. Effective intervention is particularly difficult with patients who have undergone extensive surgery, have had a limb amputated, became sterile as a result of cancer chemotherapy, or have suffered delayed puberty. Most challenging therapeutically are adolescents who have to deal with age-appropriate developmental issues that converge with cancer-related experiences. Drug compliance is a paradigm of this conflict. It means submission to and dependence upon authority, as well as inability to deny the gravity of the condition and its potential outcome. This issue was epitomized by a 15-year-old patient with non–Hodgkin's lymphoma. She resolved this conflict in an ambivalent, characteristically adolescent fashion. She would take a vial filled with the daily amount of medication and twirl it on the floor. The pills that spilled on the floor were discarded, those that stayed in the vial were taken. Based on our observations, we were able to recommend to the pediatric oncologists to refrain from asking, "Do you take your medication?" and to ask, instead, "How many pills do you throw out?" This open recognition of the way an adolescent experiences the disease makes for establishing a more honest communication between doctor and teenage patient.

Among adolescents, the fear of confronting limitations following extensive surgery (like amputation or knee replacement) can often impede recovery. Clinically it can manifest itself through pain, withdrawal, refusal, and avoidance of active participation in physiotherapy. By contrast, some teenagers attempt to engage in almost total denial of the handicap. One 17-year-old patient with osteosarcoma began daredevil stunts on motorcycles following amputation of a leg. Another patient attempted breakdancing on one leg. The risk, especially in teenage boys, is that such denial runs a thin boundary between life-threatening risk taking and successful adaptation.

It's noteworthy to mention a particular instance of acting-out in an adolescent girl. Having been told that chemotherapy might have made her sterile she became extremely sexually active—without the use of contraception. After six months she became pregnant and immediately secured an abortion. The frenetic quality of her sexual behavior evaporated once she proved she was fertile. Her own observation was, "I guess doctors aren't always right."

We find that, unless there has been excessive psychopathology prior to the occurrence of cancer, short-term crisis-oriented therapy is an accepted modality for the young patient. It does not convey the connotation of psychiatric illness, and at the same time it leaves sufficient therapeutic impact. Integrated early, it is regarded as just another element of cancer treatment.

CONCLUSION

During the past five years, our experience, in treating young cancer patients who undergo the rigors of modern cancer therapy, suggests that post-traumatic stress disorders accompanied, almost without exception, the diagnosis of childhood cancer. These observations lead us to the conclusion that it is imperative for anyone who comes in contact with the child with cancer to acknowledge the existence of, and understand the symptoms and the psychodynamics of, this diagnostic entity. Early recognition and intervention might allow for prevention of the development of the undesirable and often-severe symptoms of PTSD, a condition that can negatively affect the patient, even endangering recovery from the life-threatening disease. As we have reported elsewhere (Nir and Maslin 1982), the pediatric oncologist plays a pivotal role in the life of the young cancer patient not only due to his or her medical skills, but also because of the pediatric oncologist's central role in the management of the psychological parameters of this overwhelming medical condition. We feel that it is important to increase the effectiveness of pediatric oncologists by enabling them to attain psychotherapeutic skills. These can help physicians and their patients to negotiate the vicissitudes of the illness, from its onset, through the many remissions and relapses, and not-infrequently, death. We are currently concentrating our efforts on teaching pediatric oncologists, fellows, and residents skills that will enable them to make an early diagnosis of parental and patient coping styles, and to detect high-risk families. Another important area is the early recognition of depression in children with cancer; the most pathological manifestation of PTSD. We see the role of the liaison psychiatrist in an oncology service as primarily that of an educator and facilitator, with direct psychiatric services being provided only to patients with severe psychopathology.

REFERENCES

American Psychiatric Association: Diagnostic and Statistical Manual of Mental Disorders, 3rd ed. Washington, DC, American Psychiatric Association, 1980

Koocher GP, O'Malley JE: The Damocles Syndrome. New York, McGraw-Hill, 1981

Lazarus RS: Cognitive and coping processes in emotion, in Stress and Coping. New York, Columbia University Press, 1977

Nir Y: Psychologic support for children with soft-tissue and bone sarcomas. Proceedings of the Symposium of Sarcomas of Soft Tissue and Bone in Childhood, Orlando, Fla, 1979

Nir Y, Maslin B: Liaison Psychiatry in Childhood Cancer—A Systems Approach. Psychiatric Clinics of North America. Philadelphia, WB Saunders Co, 1982

Tamaroff M, Salwen R, Miller DR, et al: Immediate and long-term post-therapy neuropsychologic performance in children with acute lymphoblastic leukemia treated without central nervous system radiation. J Pediatr 101:524–529, 1982

Tan CTC, Tamaroff M, Nir Y, et al: Expectations and final reactions of parents of children on investigational chemotherapy, in Proceedings of the 15th annual conference of la Societé Internationale de l'Oncologie Pediatrique, York, England, 1983

Chapter 7

Children Traumatized by Physical Abuse

Arthur H. Green, M.D.

Chapter 7

Children Traumatized by Physical Abuse

The purpose of this chapter is to describe the various traumatic components of the child-abuse syndrome and to explore their impact on the growth and development of its young victims. Simultaneously, studies of abused children might provide a fertile testing ground for our theoretical formulations regarding trauma, which have been largely drawn from retrospective studies of early adverse experiences in adults. The hypotheses presented here are based upon in-depth clinical studies of approximately 50 abused children, and their families, receiving help at specialized treatment programs at the Downstate and Columbia Presbyterian Medical Centers.

Data regarding the children were obtained during their involvement in psychotherapy and play therapy. An additional 30 abused infants and preschool children were studied in the therapeutic nursery at Babies' Hospital. The setting of the nursery provided an opportunity to study the interaction between these preschoolers and their abusive parents. About 20 percent of the children were first seen during their hospitalization for their inflicted injuries. The demographic characteristics of the sample revealed that 65 percent of the children were Black, 25 percent Hispanic, and 10 percent White. The vast majority of the children resided in the inner city and lived in one-parent families. Only 20 percent lived in intact families, and almost one-half had been removed from home for at least one period in their lives.

COMPONENTS OF THE CHILD-ABUSE SYNDROME

Child abuse can be best understood as the repeated infliction of physical and psychological injury on a child by a parent within the context of a pathological parent-child and family relationship.

The immediate component, (*a*) the physical and psychological assault, is superimposed upon (*b*) a long-term harsh and punitive

135

child-rearing climate accompanied by a lack of empathic parenting; physical abuse of the child may be complicated by (c) central nervous system (CNS) impairment, which can either be a consequence of head trauma or may antedate the abuse. In the latter case, the CNS pathology may be associated with perinatal trauma or inadequate prenatal or infant care.

Acute Physical and Psychological Assault

The actual or threatened acute physical and psychological assault may create a *traumatic neurosis*, a situation that results in ego disorganization, narcissistic injury, and a painful affective state, which, in turn, activate primitive defense mechanisms and a compulsion to repeat the trauma.

It is hard to imagine anything more terrifying to an infant or young child than to be punched, kicked, burned, or hurled across a room without warning by an uncontrolled parental figure from whom nurturance and protection are usually expected. Most of the abused children perceived this type of abuse as a danger to their physical and psychological integrity. They felt threatened with annihilation and/or abandonment. They were often overwhelmed by the quantity and quality of the noxious stimulation, and by the accompanying painful affective state which paralyzed ego functions and resulted in severe panic.

The assault could not be adequately processed or controlled by the young victim's defensive organization. The child's feelings of helplessness and panic were often accompanied by a severe ego regression, characterized by (a) loss of ego boundaries, (b) psychotic disorganization, and (c) a suspension of reality testing.

> Doris, an 11-year-old girl, had been subjected to harsh beatings by her rigid, fanatically religious mother, who was impatient with Doris's failure to perform chores and errands efficiently. Once Doris tried to run away from this irate woman, who chased her with a strap after she accidentally spilled the contents of a package she was carrying. When her mother finally cornered her in the bedroom, Doris panicked and jumped out of the window. She miraculously survived the fall with only a broken femur. Her play included repetitive themes of children fleeing various monsters and killers. She described frequent nightmares and slept poorly.

Since we are often unable to observe these children immediately after the actual assault, we often fail to appreciate the true nature of their panic and anguish. Typically, the child arrives at the hospital hours or even days after the beating, with demeanor usually subdued and affect constricted, indicating the onset of defensive operations.

Primitive Defense Mechanisms

Primitive defense mechanisms were usually employed by the abused children in attempting to control repeated traumatic overstimulation and accompanying painful affects. They used defensive operations such as avoidance and distancing behavior, raising of sensory thresholds, denial, projection, and splitting. These defenses were often reinforced by the pervasive denial of the ideational and affective impact of the abusive incidents. This suppression of the perception of parental assault was occasionally motivated by parental threats of additional punishment, but it also was associated with the children's desperate need to protect themselves from the terrifying awareness of the parents' destructive impulses toward them, the acknowledgment of which reality would lead to fears of annihilation and/or intense retaliatory rage, which would endanger the child's psychological survival.

Avoidance and Distancing Behavior. Abused infants and toddlers observed in the hospital or therapeutic nursery frequently displayed avoidance and distancing behaviors as a means of protection against the frightening parent. They often avoided eye contact, which might have originated in gaze aversion during infancy, which could be regarded as a primordial defense against noxious stimulation. Some infants and toddlers exhibited the symptom of *frozen watchfulness*, described by Ounstead et al. (1974). They sat passively and immobile, but were alert and hypervigilant so as to detect possible danger in the environment. George and Main (1979) observed that abused toddlers tended to avoid their mothers, even when they made friendly overtures. When they did respond, they approached them to the side, or to the rear, or by back-stepping. Abused toddlers in the hospital or nursery often preferred to attach themselves to unfamiliar staff members, while turning away from their parents. These symptoms of visual avoidance, hypervigilance, and extreme wariness in the presence of a caretaker perceived to be harmful might represent precursors of paranoid and projective defenses appearing later in childhood.

This defensive adaptation to the abusive environment produces additional sequelae. When receptor functions ordinarily available for processing the environment are overinvolved in identifying potential danger, learning becomes compromised. Twenty-five percent of our sample of 60 abused children of school age evaluated at the Downstate Medical Center were found to be mentally retarded, with IQs of less than 70 (Sandgrund et al. 1974). Similar intellectual impairment in abused children was described by Martin et al. (1974) and

Morse et al. (1970). The hypervigilant defenses are also associated with inhibitions of speech and motility, which appear to be a consequence of learned avoidance. For example, abused infants and toddlers are frequently beaten when they cry or vocalize for attention. They eventually learn to curb their verbal expressiveness in the interest of self-preservation. Speech and language disorders have been commonly observed in follow-up studies of abused children (Martin 1972; Elmer and Gregg 1967; and Kempe 1976).

Denial, Projection, and Splitting. The perception of parental malevolence was frequently denied by the children and displaced onto some other person, or themselves. This allowed the child to maintain the fantasy of having a "good parent." This parental splitting was associated with a corresponding splitting of the self-representation into "good" and "bad" components. Splitting mechanisms were more frequently and dramatically present in those children whose abusive parents were their sole caretakers.

Repetition of the Trauma

The primitive defensive operations previously described were usually not successful in binding the anxiety generated by the repeated physical assault. The original traumatic imagery derived from the beatings permeated the dreams, fantasies, play, and object relationships of the abused children. During their reenactment of the trauma during play therapy and psychotherapy, the children conveyed their helplessness and sense of being overwhelmed. At times they viewed themselves as passive victims, but on other occasions in fantasy or in play with peers, they tended actively to repeat the original traumatic situation by attacking and injuring others, so as to emulate the parent aggressor (see case illustration on Juan). Some of the children perpetuated the trauma by engaging in self-destructive activity or accident-proneness, or attempted to provoke physical attack from the environment.

> Sarah, age six, had been a victim of recurrent physical abuse by her mother since infancy. She sustained a broken femur following a severe beating when she was four. On this occasion her mother attacked her for letting the bathroom sink overflow. During her initial testing, Sarah responded to the examiner's presentation of a hitting scene in a doll family with the comment: "The mother hits the baby for playing with water." During the psychiatric interview a short time later, Sarah appeared quite anxious upon returning from the bathroom. She told the psychiatrist that she was afraid he would punish her for spilling water from the sink onto the floor.

The "fixation" persisted throughout our contact with these children, despite the cessation of physical abuse as a result of therapeutic intervention with the families. Repetition of the trauma was incited by situations that threatened the child's safety and self-esteem. Rejections, humiliations, and physical confrontations were consciously or unconsciously linked to the original parental abuse and scapegoating, and resulted in a narcissistic injury and/or threat of annihilation.

Repetition of the trauma may also be regarded as a primitive defense mechanism, in which the traumatic elements are reenacted in a relatively unmodified form in an attempt to achieve mastery over a passively experienced danger. The child tries to recreate, master, and control painful affects and anxiety initiated during the abusive experience.

Long-Term Traumatic Elements

The following types of chronic parental dysfunction exert a cumulative and noxious impact on the child's ego functioning and development. They are consistent with Khan's (1963) concept of *cumulative trauma* caused by the mother's failure to function as a protective

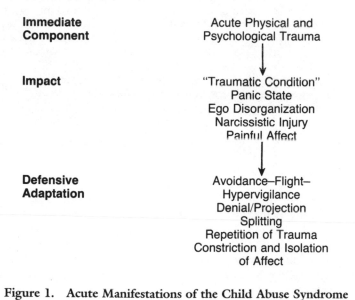

Immediate Component	Acute Physical and Psychological Trauma
Impact	"Traumatic Condition" Panic State Ego Disorganization Narcissistic Injury Painful Affect
Defensive Adaptation	Avoidance–Flight– Hypervigilance Denial/Projection Splitting Repetition of Trauma Constriction and Isolation of Affect

Figure 1. Acute Manifestations of the Child Abuse Syndrome

shield, and Kris's (1956) notion of a *strain trauma*, which refers to the traumatic effects of long-lasting situations.

Harsh and Punitive Child Rearing. Early exposure of an infant to a harsh and punitive parental figure promotes primary identification with the aggressive parent. *Identification with the aggressor* is used as a major defense mechanism in situations of anxiety provoked by fears of attack, humiliation, and abandonment. This defense permits the child's fears of helplessness and annihilation to be replaced by feelings of power and omnipotence.

> Juan, an 11-year-old boy, was referred for psychiatric treatment after he persuaded his 3-year-old half brother to drink some lye. One year prior to this incident, Juan had returned to live with his mother and her boyfriend after having spent the previous 7 years with his physically abusive father and stepmother in Puerto Rico. Juan had been subjected to chronic physical abuse during this period, which consisted of beatings on the head and burns on his body inflicted with a hot iron. Since living with his mother, Juan displayed hyperactive, aggressive behavior in school, frequently hitting and kicking his classmates. He had also demonstrated extreme jealousy of his two younger half brothers, encountered for the first time. He had teased and attacked them since his return home. Juan disclosed to his therapist that he enjoyed catching mice and smashing their heads with a hammer. He would then flush them down the toilet. When asked to explain the reasons for this behavior, Juan pointed to the scars and ridges on his scalp exclaiming, "This is what my father did to me!"

In children like Juan, aggressive and assaultive behavior become the primary vehicle for establishing object ties.

The compulsive, repetitive quality of the aggressive and violent interactions of these abused children suggests that identification with the aggressor is also used as a device for relieving tension, counteracting painful affects, and as a pathological form of self-esteem regulation.

This aggressive adaptation to danger has also been observed in maltreated infants and toddlers. George and Main (1979) reported assaultive behavior in abused children from one to three years of age in a day care setting. These children frequently hit or threatened the staff members. Fraiberg (1982) observed the same phenomenon in infants subjected to danger and deprivation. She conceptualized this "fighting" as a pathological pre-ego defense against the danger of helplessness and self-dissolution.

Longitudinal observations of these aggressive responses in abused infants and toddlers suggest that the early (and predominately imitative) patterns of aggression become transformed gradually into the more highly structured identification with the aggressor with the growth of ego development and ego differentiation.

Scapegoating. Physical abuse and mental cruelty are often directed to one child in a family. This scapegoated child is blamed for the shortcomings and inadequacy of the parents and siblings. This child is the one most closely identified with the abusing parent, reminding the parent of his or her own unacceptable traits and impulses. These parental deficiencies are projected onto the child, who, being unaware of the distorting nature of the scapegoating process, assumes that he or she is to blame and is deserving of the punishment. This increases self-hatred, low self-esteem, and depressive affect. This introjection of the parental hostility and rejection becomes the nucleus of a punitive superego and subsequent self-destructive behavior. In fact, 40 percent of our research sample of 60 abused children evaluated at the Downstate Medical Center exhibited self-destructive behavior, which included suicidal gestures and attempts, suicidal ideation, and self-mutilation (Green 1978b). Even abused and neglected toddlers have been observed to turn aggression against themselves (Fraiberg 1982). These self-destructive behaviors represent the children's conscious or unconscious compliance with parental wishes for their destruction and/or disappearance. The child's acting-out of parental hostility directed towards him or her has been described by Sabbeth (1969) as an important factor in the etiology of adolescent suicidal behavior. The transformation of the abused child's self-hatred into self-destructive behavior is catalyzed by poor impulse control and a defect in the ego functions mediating self-preservation. Khantzian and Mack (1983) regard the capacity for self-care and self-preservation as an ego function, originating in the internalization of the protective qualities of the parents, which is closely associated with positive self-esteem. The ego's regulation of self-preservation is obviously undermined in an abusive caretaking environment. The self-destructive impact of an abusive parental introject is illustrated by the following case:

Betty, an eight-year-old girl had been abused by her impulsive alcoholic mother. The beatings were often triggered by the mother's heavy drinking. When Betty was seven, she jumped off a swing in response to the commands of a "woman's voice," and sustained a fractured arm. She was also severely accident-prone. Some of her typical comments during her psychotherapy sessions were: "My mother says I'm terrible because I can't sit still. I'm always hurting myself. I fall off my bike and lean against a hot radiator." When she was angry with her therapist, or her mother, she would often bang her arm or head against a hard object, stick herself with a pin, or threaten to jump out of the window.

In the majority of cases, the self-destructive behavior was precipitated by parental beatings or by threatened or actual separation from parental figures.

A majority of the abused children displayed provocative pain-seeking behavior, whether or not they were overtly self-destructive. They frequently provoked arguments and fights with siblings, peers, and authority figures, in addition to their own abusing parents. When abused children are placed into foster homes, they often provoke beatings from foster parents. Their pain-dependent and self-defeating behavior is quite different from that of the "guilt-ridden" masochistic character. It does not appear to be motivated by unconscious guilt or related to psychic conflict. Its roots seem to originate in the earliest traumatic encounters with abusing primary objects during infancy and early childhood and it serves a defensive function for the children in the context of a traumatic environment. For example, by provoking a potentially abusive parent, the child achieves a sense of mastery by controlling the timing and perhaps the intensity of the beating. There is time to take defensive action while bracing oneself for the attack. This alleviates the much greater fear of being attacked and overwhelmed unexpectedly and without warning. In other words, signal anxiety is invoked to prevent traumatic anxiety.

Provocation of abuse from the parent also provides the child who is otherwise neglected and understimulated with physical contact and attention, which is usually unavailable.

Maternal Deprivation and Family Disorganization. Child abuse occurring in multiproblem, impoverished families is often associated with other types of parental dysfunction such as neglect, multiple caretaking, maternal deprivation, and substandard physical care. Defects in parenting are often compounded by a highly stressful environment and lack of support systems. The children in these families are frequently exposed to separations from primary objects during their early years.

The abuse itself often results in temporary or long-term placement of the children in foster homes or institutions. Thus, the detrimental effects of deprivation and neglect (such as apathy, withdrawal, cognitive impairment, affect hunger with superficiality of object relations, low frustration tolerance, lack of basic trust, impaired object constancy, and faulty superego development) will be superimposed upon the sequelae of physical abuse. It is often difficult to isolate the impact of abuse in children who are also neglected. In fact, our population of neglected, nonabused children at Downstate Medical Center demonstrated the same degree of cognitive impairment as the abused sample (Sandgrund et al. 1974).

Some of the abused children often reacted to threatened and actual separation and object loss with intense anxiety. This seemed related to their inability to achieve object constancy as a result of frequent early experiences of abandonment and separation. The lack of object constancy was also influenced by the presence of cognitive impairment and/or cerebral dysfunction, which interfered with the construction and internalization of the absent object. This was frequently observed in the treatment situation in response to termination of contact with the therapist. Many of the children had difficulty handling the routine separation at the end of their treatment hour, as evidenced by their reluctance to leave the playroom. Acute separation anxiety and panic states were often observed in response to the therapist's vacations and departure from the hospital.

Defenses Against Painful Affects

The painful affects and impaired self-concept resulting from the immediate and long-term traumatic components of the child-abuse syndrome constitute a severe narcissistic injury for the children which, in turn, generates additional defensive activity. The abused children gradually increased their tolerance for painful affects with the passage of time. The intensity of their initial fears of annihilation, abandonment, and feelings of helplessness were eventually dampened by a gradual constriction of affect. These children eventually described the frightening details of their batterings in a bland and detached manner. They often smiled as they recounted specific memories of their beatings. Defenses of denial, isolation, and constriction of affect offered them further protection from these traumatic memories. Reexperiencing these painful emotions would have constituted an additional trauma for these children. "Grown-up," formerly abused children display this numbing of affect as they smile while describing the beneficial effects of their beatings, which they use to rationalize their current use of violent corporal punishment. Unfortunately, this rigid defensive posture makes it impossible for them to empathize with the suffering of their own children.

As the scapegoated children grow older, they attempt to transfer their negative self-image to others by means of projection and externalization. Unfortunately, their own children ultimately become the recipients of this displacement, and the cycle of scapegoating and abuse repeats itself in the next generation.

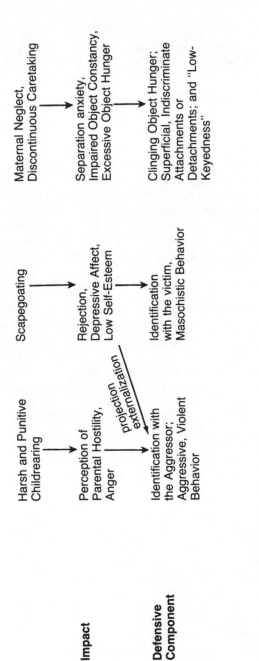

Figure 2. Long-Term Traumatic Elements

Central Nervous System Impairment

Martin et al. (1974) and Green et al. (1981) detected a high incidence of neurological abnormalities in abused children, many of whom had no history of head trauma. Neurological damage may result from injury to the child's brain as a consequence of direct trauma to the head (skull fracture, cerebral hemorrhage), or indirect trauma such as the *shaking injury* described by Caffey (1972), in which violent shaking of a baby's head can produce petechial hemorrhages in brain tissue. Sandgrund et al. (1974) described a high incidence of mental retardation in a population of abused children who had no evidence of head trauma. We concluded that, in many of these children, the prior brain damage and retardation might be regarded as a cause of rather than a consequence of physical abuse.

Regardless of the etiology, a child with neurological impairment will be more vulnerable to the traumatic impact of physical abuse. The CNS impairment in itself will further undermine the cognitive, adaptive, and defensive functions of the ego during their response to trauma, and will facilitate the direct expression of impulse.

RETRAUMATIZATION

Once the child has experienced the overwhelming anxiety and painful affects associated with the traumatic event, he or she remains in constant dread of its recurrence. In a hypervigilant state, he or she is extremely sensitive to external events which might resemble the trauma in any way. These traumatic "signals" can trigger the circumvention of the old feelings of helplessness and panic by initiating defensive activity. The child is ready for "fight or flight," depending on the circumstances. Unfortunately, these emergency responses become overgeneralized, and may occur in situations in which there is no objective danger. This very anticipation of the trauma might be as traumatic as the original event. Thus the internal stimuli or events, in the form of fantasies and memories of the attack, can impinge on the stimulus barrier and cause as much distress as the beatings themselves. The child's fear of further attack is similar to Rado's (1942) concept of traumatophobia, applied to victims of traumatic war neuroses. They were incapacitated by their memories of combat, as the threats of war were extended to all prospective dangers in civilian life. If the child's defensive actions result in a successful avoidance or attenuation of the physical assault, some degree of mastery and reduction of anxiety may be achieved. If the battering continues in an unpredictable fashion despite all defensive efforts, the child will be traumatized by both the noxious external stimulation and its internalized representations. Breaching of the stimulus barrier will ensue, leading to a full-blown traumatic neurosis and collapse of ego functioning. At this point, the child might develop panic states, psychotic disorganization, psychosomatic symptoms, or a depressive withdrawal. When the battering results in bodily injury, further dimensions of trauma are added. Physical suffering is superimposed upon the psychological pain. If hospitalization is required, the child experiences additional separation anxiety, object loss, and the trauma of painful medical surgical procedures.

Long-Term Traumatic Effects

The cumulative impact of the repeated physical assaults, inflicted on a background of harsh and punitive caretaking, scapegoating, and deprivation exerts a detrimental effect on the future psychological adaptation of the abused child. The defensive maneuvers which "protected" the helpless child within the traumatic environment persist into adulthood, where the internalized battleground of childhood is perpetually recreated with new objects in a new setting. The hypervigilant, frozen, mistrustful child is often transformed into the suspicious, hypersensitive adult paranoid. Failure to master the trauma of childhood creates a continual need to repeat and reenact them during adult life. Through the use of identification with the aggressor, violent assaultive behavior is utilized as an adaptive response to potentially dangerous situations that are unconsciously linked to the original abuse. However, the connection between the present and past dangers is obliterated by the persisting repression and constriction and isolation of affect. The assaultive behavior is also used for tension release and as a pathological form of self-esteem regulation. Aggressor–victim relationships become the norm, based upon the internalized "angry parent–bad child" images from the past. These individuals are distrustful in the presence of nonthreatening individuals, and seek to restore the familiar sadomasochistic interaction by engaging in provocative behavior, thus protecting themselves against possible betrayal and rationalizing their continued defensive use of aggression. Some formerly abused adults cling to their identification with the victim, and perpetuate their pain-dependent defensive style. We often see this in abused girls who become repeatedly pregnant as teenagers by assaultive boyfriends, modeled after their abusing parents. Unfortunately for their children, they step out of the victim role after their babies are born, and proceed to abuse them, identifying with their own abusing parents. It is common for some of these women to deploy identification with the aggressor and identification with the victim simultaneously, in the roles of abusing mother and battered spouse. Aside from the pathological object relationship and deviant parenting just outlined, additional long-term sequelae include cognitive impairment and vocational failure, crime and delinquency, chronic depression with anhedonia, and severe borderline and narcissistic pathology.

The following case history will illustrate the relationship between early exposure to severe abuse and deviant child rearing, and the subsequent development of pathological defenses with violent life-threatening behavior.

Charles, a black youth, currently 16 years of age, was born when his mother Sally was 13. She had been living with a female cousin and the cousin's husband when Charles was conceived. Sally had been beaten by her cousin and repeatedly sexually abused by the cousin's husband since she was sent to live with them at the age of 4, when her mother died. When Charles was born, Sally lived alone in a room and lacked the money to adequately feed and clothe him. She initially regarded the baby as "unreal, like a doll" and expected that he would make her happy. However, when he cried out of hunger, she beat him "so he would shut up and go to sleep. I beat him so long he'd be crazy," Sally confessed. "I hit him with a belt, extension cord, and anything I could get my hands on."

Charles lived with his mother until he was 4, and was then sent to his maternal aunt for 2 years. After this, he was shifted back and forth between his mother, his aunt, and his maternal grandfather in Florida. He was returned to his mother, now living in New York, at the age of 16, after he was placed on probation for shooting his junior high school teacher with a pellet gun. This incident occurred after he was reprimanded by the teacher for fighting with a classmate. After the teacher hit him in front of the class, Charles announced that he would return with a gun and take revenge. He carried out the threat and proceeded to shoot the teacher in the leg. After his return to New York, Charles continued to experience difficulties in school. He was also abusive to his younger brother and was involved in stealing. Another violent incident occurred when Charles shot a gun into a crowd of hostile white youths who were taunting him and several of his friends after a rock concert. Luckily, no one was hit, and Charles was arrested on the spot. Charles had obtained the gun by stealing it from his friend's father, and carried it with him in anticipation of an attack. He seemed unperturbed when confronted with the possibility that he might have injured or killed someone, blandly responding, "If somebody got killed, he deserved it." His principal hobbies and interests are guns and vicious dogs. He is fascinated with bull terriers because they can be trained to keep potential attackers at bay, and kill them if necessary. In a recurrent fantasy, his bull terrier carries out his command to kill an intruder. When he becomes 18, he plans to join the army and become a "ranger," to receive training in special gun tactics. He would like to be a sniper, so he can stalk his enemies at a distance, and then shoot them. Charles experiences frequent violent nightmares, the most recent depicting his friend trying to kill him.

From the data presented thus far, it would appear that most abused children are destined to become severely damaged adults, most likely to repeat their traumatic experiences with others, including their own children. However, at child-abuse treatment programs, we do not encounter the formerly abused individuals who become good parents, striving to protect their children from the harm that they experienced. But these people do exist. They may be spared from a life focused on violent expectations and defensive aggression because of the availability of a gentle, nonpunitive parental figure during childhood, who served as a benign model for identification. Or, perhaps, they possessed intrinsic ego strength, which provided them with a tool for mastery. However, despite a "normal" facade, these individuals must wage a constant struggle to defend themselves against the painful memories of childhood trauma, pent-up rage, and negative self and object representations, which threaten to engulf them.

Diagnostic Considerations

About one-half of the abused children encountered in our treatment program satisfy the *Diagnostic and Statistical Manual* of Mental Disorders (*DSM-III*, American Psychiatric Press 1980) diagnostic criteria for post-traumatic stress disorder (PTSD) in that:

1. The acute and long-term traumatic components of the child-abuse syndrome constitute recognizable stressors.
2. Reexperiencing of the trauma, as evidenced by recurrent dreams and intrusive recollections of the parental violence and hostility
3. Reduced involvement with the external world, manifested by signs of detachment and prominent constriction of affect
4. The following symptoms were often manifested as sequelae of the abuse: hypervigilance, sleep disturbance, avoidance of activities or situations which might result in retraumatization, and intensification of symptoms (i.e., hyperaggressive, pain-dependent, or phobic behavior during exposure to events which symbolize or resemble the abusive situation).

The fear of retraumatization may produce an exacerbation of an acute post-traumatic stress disorder in a formerly abused child who previously appeared to be asymptomatic or afflicted with a chronic post-traumatic stress disorder.

Abused children display a wide variety of other psychiatric diagnoses, which may or may not be related to their traumatization. The most frequent Axis I diagnoses accompanying the PTSD are conduct disorders, anxiety disorders, dysthymic disorder, and specific developmental disorders listed on Axis II.

IMPACT ON TRAUMA THEORY

One might apply Freud's concepts of traumatic neurosis and the stimulus barrier, described in *Beyond the Pleasure Principle* (1920) and *Inhibitions, Symptoms, and Anxiety* (1926), to the acute traumatic situation resulting from child abuse. Freud regarded the infant's high threshold for the perception of stimuli as a protective shield, or stimulus barrier. He described as *traumatic* any excitation powerful enough to break through the protective shield. The traumatic situation was defined as the experience of helplessness on the part of the ego in the face of accumulation of excitation, whether of external or internal origin. The pleasure principle is put out of action, and a regression ensues in which primitive modes of functioning are utilized in order to master and bind the stimulus. The repetition compulsion, or need to repeat painful traumatic events, was ultimately regarded as a manifestation of the death instinct, or primary masochism. Freud distinguished between signal anxiety, the ego's response to the threat of danger, and automatic anxiety, the reaction to the situation of helplessness experienced during the traumatic situation. In *Moses and Monotheism* (1939), Freud noted the importance of the interaction between constitutional factors and experiences, and contrasted the positive and negative effects of traumas. Positive effects are described as attempts to repeat the painful trauma, while negative effects are defensive reactions designed to avoid the traumatic experience. Freud postulated that both the positive and negative reactions represent fixations to the trauma.

Most recent observations of children have broadened the concept of trauma to include adverse conditions that do not involve a breakthrough of the stimulus barrier and an ensuing state of helplessness. Kris proposed the term strain trauma to describe the effect of longlasting situations that cause traumatic effects by the accumulation of frustrating tensions. Khan (1963) stressed the mother's role as a protective shield and auxiliary ego for the vulnerable infant. The mother's failure to carry out this protective role may lead to widespread deficits in ego functioning on the basis of cumulative trauma, which becomes visible only in retrospect. According to Khan, the cumulative trauma builds up silently throughout childhood up to adolescence. Boyer (1956) also described the mother's role as a supplementary stimulus barrier and cited her potential to traumatize the infant through overstimulation. Winnicott (1960) referred to the mother's protective role as the *good-enough* holding environment, which is necessary for optimal ego development. These broader categories of trauma resulting from pathological parenting have been rejected by some (Freud 1967; Rangell 1967; and Krystal 1978) for being too general. They regard the overwhelming of the ego, with the release of painful affects, as the essential components of trauma. Greenacre (1967) favors a wider definition of trauma that includes any conditions that seem unfavorable, noxious, or drastically injurious to the development of the young individual. This concept of trauma encompasses both the immediate and the cumulative subtypes.

In the child-abuse syndrome, the abusing parent abrogates his or her role as a protective shield and, additionally, floods the child with acute painful physical and psychological stimulation, within the context of a long-term mutually frustrating relationship that fails to satisfy the basic psychological needs of the child. Neither the acute nor the long-term traumatic elements, alone, can account for the widespread disorder of ego functions, object relations, and affective regulations which ensue. It is more parsimonious to visualize an interactive potentiating effect between these types of trauma, in which the long-standing impact of both the shock and the cumulative traumas render the ego more vulnerable to subsequent shock traumas of physical assault.

Freud's model of the protective shield, or stimulus barrier, does not adequately describe the complex mechanisms involved in the processing of external and internal stimuli. Freud regarded the stimulus barrier as an essentially passive mechanism: a physical barrier or threshold which tended to reduce levels of stimulation. Freud felt that the stimulus barrier was exclusively directed against external stimuli. Observations of abused children, however, suggest that they defend themselves simultaneously against both the external traumatic stimulation and its internal reverberations. This stimulus-barrier function of the ego is achieved through active defensive efforts.

I would suggest that the so-called breaching of the stimulus barrier could be more aptly described as a damaging of the ego structures involved in the reception, processing, and integration of stimuli, by the shocking traumatic events. The resulting sensory overload, in turn, gives rise to the raising of sensory thresholds, evidenced by defensive activity dominated by hypervigilance and avoidance. The associated painful mental imagery is controlled by denial, repression, projection, and constriction of affect. These defensive efforts fail when the impact of the trauma damages the protective and receptive functions of the ego beyond a critical point. The damaged or weakened ego then resorts to a driven, compulsive repetition and reenactment of the traumatic elements. Greenacre (1967) regarded the very young child (infancy through 28 months) as particularly vulnerable to trauma, which might leave an organized imprint on the child that, in turn, could induce a greater need for repetition.

Our observations of abused children in the nursery and playroom settings reveal that, at times, these reenactments often intensified their anxiety instead of containing it. This could confirm Terr's (1981) thesis that post-traumatic play is ineffective because the child's identifications with the violent aggressor or helpless victim are too frightening to permit the gaining of enough emotional disturbance from the traumatic event. The repetition compulsion, then, may be regarded as the ego's last line of defense against traumatic stimulation. Its success or failure to achieve mastery will depend on the strength of the ego, in relation to the magnitude of the traumatic event. This model of trauma is consistent with Benjamin's (1965) and Bellak's (1973) concept of the stimulus barrier as an active, adaptive ego function, and Brody and Axelrad's (1966) view of the receptive and integrative functions of the protective shield.

The pathological impact of cumulative trauma would be primarily exerted upon the child's affective development, and on ego functions involving self-preservation and the establishment of object relationships and identifications. Cumulative trauma would also adversely affect the long-term shaping of ego defenses, determining character formation, and would interfere with mastery and cognitive development. Since the pathological impact of cumulative trauma is exerted gradually, it will have a less dramatic effect on the receptive ego functions.

IMPLICATIONS FOR TREATMENT

Intervention with abusing parents and amelioration of the abusive environment, although necessary for the child's welfare, are not sufficient to reverse the victim's ego impairment and the pathological personality changes resulting from the traumatic components of the abuse. Many of the defensive maneuvers designed to reestablish ego integrity and affective equilibrium, and to ward off further assault, are distinctly maladaptive in nontraumatic environments.

A wide range of psychotherapeutic and educational techniques have proven successful in alleviating the symptoms and distress experienced by the abused children. Psychoanalytically oriented play therapy and psychotherapy have been used effectively in our treatment programs (Green, 1978a). Certain modifications of therapeutic techniques are necessary to deal with the high incidence of ego deviation, cognitive impairment, impulsivity, and pathological object relations and identifications. The abused children often require the type of environmental manipulation and structuring employed with borderline and psychotic children. Their deprivation and maltreatment by primary objects justifies a more-supportive and flexible therapeutic stance, with some gratification of their dependency needs. Strengthening of ego functions becomes a major focus, with an emphasis on reality testing, increasing frustration tolerance, and encouraging verbalization as an alternative to the repetitive physical reenactment of traumatic events as the major mode of expression. Higher-level defenses, such as repression and sublimation, are strengthened, in order to replace primitive mechanisms of denial, projection, splitting, and identification with the aggressor. Impulsive and aggressive outbursts in the playroom must be actively curtailed. Consolidation of the therapeutic alliance facilitates a gradual internalization of the therapist's superego structure and controls, and permits the modification of pathological self and object representations. Psychoeducational intervention can be employed to deal with learning difficulties based upon cognitive and attentional deficits. In the absence of intervention, abused children are vulnerable to subsequent psychological impairment, vocational and educational failure, violence, delinquency, and criminality, and are likely to repeat the patterns of maltreatment with their own children.

SUMMARY

This chapter describes the various traumatic components of the child-abuse syndrome and explores their impact on the psychopathology, cognitive impairment, and developmental sequelae observed in abused children. The child-abuse syndrome consists of two main categories of trauma: The acute physical and psychological assault confronting the child with the threat of annihilation is superimposed upon the long-term traumatic components resulting from chronic abnormal parenting, such as harsh, punitive child rearing, scapegoating, and maternal deprivation. Central nervous system impairment, which is frequently associated with child abuse, may be regarded as an additional source of trauma which potentiates the pathological impact of the acute and long-term components of the abusive environment. Many abused children exhibit the characteristic symptoms of PTSD.

It is hypothesized that the acute trauma might damage ego structures involved in the reception, processing, and integration of stimuli, which contributes to the repetition and reenactment of the traumatic event. The pathological impact of the long-term traumatic events are most likely exerted on the child's affective development, and ego functions involving self-preservation and the establishment of object relationships and identifications.

REFERENCES

American Psychiatric Association: Diagnostic and Statistical Manual of Mental Disorders, 3rd ed. Washington, DC, American Psychiatric Association, 1980

Bellak L, Hurvich M, Gediman H: Ego Functions in Schizophrenics, Neurotics, and Normals. New York, John Wiley & Sons, 1973

Benjamin J: Developmental biology and psychoanalysis, in Psychoanalysis and Current Biological Thought. Edited by Greenfield N, Lewis W. Madison, University of Wisconsin, 1965, pp 57–80

Boyer LB: On maternal overstimulation and ego defects. Psychoanal Study Child 11:236–256, 1956

Brody S, Axelrad S: Anxiety, socialization, and ego formation in infancy. Int J Psychoanal 47:218–229, 1966

Caffey J: On the theory and practice of shaking infants: its potential residual effects of permanent damage and mental retardation. Am J Dis Child 124:160–161, 1972

Elmer E, Gregg CS: Developmental characteristics of abused children. Pediatrics 40:596–602, 1967

Fraiberg S: Pathological defenses in infancy. Psychoanal Q 51:612–635, 1982

Freud A: Comments on trauma, in Psychic Trauma. Edited by Furst S. New York, Basic Books, 1967, pp 235–245

Freud S: Inhibitions, symptoms, and anxiety, in The Standard Edition of the Complete Psychological Works of Sigmund Freud, vol. 18. Edited by Strachey J. London, Hogarth Press, 1926, pp 3–64

Freud S: Inhibitions, symptoms, and anxiety, in The Standard Edition of the Complete Psychological Works of Sigmund Freud, vol. 20. Edited by Strachey J. London, Hogarth Press, 1920, pp 75–175

Freud S: Moses and monotheism, in The Standard Edition of the Complete Psychological Works of Sigmund Freud, vol. 23. Edited by Strachey J. London, Hogarth Press, 1939, pp 1–137

George C, Main M: Social interactions and young abused children: Approach, avoidance, and aggression. Child Dev 50:306–319, 1979

Green AH: Psychiatric treatment of abused children. J Am Acad Child Psychiatry 17:356–371, 1978a

Green AH: Self-destructive behavior in battered children. Am J Psychiatry 135:579–582, 1978b

Greenacre P: The influence of infantile trauma on genetic patterns, in Psychic Trauma. Edited by Furst S. New York, Basic Books, 1967, pp 108–153

Kempe P: Arresting or freezing the developmental process, in Child Abuse and Neglect, the Family and Community. Edited by Helter RE, Kempe CH. Cambridge, Ballinger, 1976, pp 64–73

Khan M: The concept of cumulative trauma. Psychoanal Study Child 18:54–88, 1963

Khantzian E, Mack J: Self-preservation and care of the self: ego instincts reconsidered. Psychoanal Study Child 38:209–232, 1983

Kris E: The recovery of childhood memories. Psychoanal Study Child 11:54–88, 1956

Krystal H: Trauma and affect. Psychoanal Study Child 33:8–116, 1978

Martin HP: The child and his development, in Helping the Battered Child and His Family. Edited by Kempe CH, Helfer RE. Philadelphia, JB Lippincott Co, 1972, pp 93–114

Martin HP: The Abused Child: A Multidisciplinary Approach to Developmental Issues and Treatment. Cambridge, Ballinger, 1976

Martin HP, Breezly P, Conway EF, et al: The development of abused children. Advances in Pediatrics 21:439–447, 1974

Morse W, Sahler OJ, Friedman SB: A three-year follow-up study of abused children. Am J Dis Child 120:439–446, 1970

Ounstead C, Oppenheimer R, Lindsay J: Aspects of bonding failure: The psychotherapeutic treatment of families of battered children. Dev Med Child Neurol 16:446–456, 1974

Rado S: Psychodynamics and treatment of traumatic war neurosis (traumatophobia). Psychosomatic Medicine 4:362–368, 1942

Sabbeth J: The suicidal adolescent. J Am Acad Child Psychiatry 8:272–286, 1969

Sandgrund A, Gaines RW, Green AH: Child abuse and mental retardation: a problem of cause and effect. Am J Ment Defic 79:327–330, 1974

Terr L: 'Forbidden games': post-traumatic child's play. J Am Acad Child Psychiatry 20:741–760, 1981

Winnicott D: The theory of the parent–infant relationship, in The Maturational Processes and the Facilitating Environment. New York, International Universities Press, 1960, pp 37–55

Chapter 8

Post-Traumatic Symptoms in Incest Victims

Jean Goodwin, M.D., M.P.H.

Chapter 8

Post-Traumatic Symptoms in Incest Victims

I n 1896, Sigmund Freud reported 18 cases of hysteria; in each case, he had uncovered a history of sexual abuse in the patient's childhood. Freud found that the sexual-abuse experience could be reconstructed from the pattern of the patient's hysterical and obsessive symptoms, even when that experience had been completely repressed. Ultimately, the sexual "scenes" were relived in abreaction during psychoanalytic or hypnotherapeutic treatment, and symptoms disappeared (Masson 1984; Miller 1984).

Freud (1954) eventually renounced these findings, saying that he had been naive to mistake for actual memories the Oedipal fantasies of patients who had merely longed for sexual adventures with their parents. However, although Freud published many cases, including the famous case of Dora (Freud 1905; Erikson 1962; Balmary 1982), in which the patient's complaint about a sexually seductive adult was corroborated by other family members, he never published a case in which sexual allegations could be translated, entirely, as remembered fantasies (Goodwin et al. 1979). In the absence of clinical material one is not even certain what Freud meant by "fantasies"—screen memories, delusions, opportunistic lies, imaginary experiences of alter personalities? Nevertheless, this concept, that accounts of childhood sexual events might represent fantasies, helped delay for nearly 80 years the elaboration and replication of his original work.

The present chapter will review recent attempts to build on Freud's early ideas by tracing symptom development to childhood efforts to defend against the physical and psychosocial trauma of sexual abuse. Two basic questions have remained in dispute since Freud's first paper. First, can sexual encounters in childhood be considered as traumatic events? Second, are the victims of such experiences symptomatic, and can their symptoms be related to the sexual abuse?

Case material in this chapter will describe victims of incest, that is, individuals who were sexually exploited as children by an adult in a parental role (Goodwin 1982). Freud (1896) noted that this was the most common type of sexual abuse in his series and that this kind of abuse often led to further sexual abuse by unrelated or peer perpetrators. Several case histories of incest victims will be reviewed, in which the observed symptom pattern was similar to that described for post-traumatic disorders (PTSD) in combat veterans and in rape victims. Most incest victims who request treatment meet criteria for post-traumatic disorder, although this can be difficult to recognize, either due to the victim's young age, the severity of symptoms, or the victim's tendency to conceal both symptoms and the extent of the prior sexual abuse.

IS INCEST TRAUMATIC?

In the 1890s, Freud did not have difficulty convincing his readers that incest was a traumatic, overwhelming experience for a child. This was assumed, just as readily as it was assumed that incest occurred only rarely, one case per million population (Henderson 1975), too rarely for Freud's data to be correct. Today, as more surveys tell us that one to five percent of women in the general population have experienced incest with a father or step father (Goodwin et al. 1981), it is no longer self-evident that all such episodes must be automatically traumatizing.

In this era of social and sexual permissiveness, there is even a pro-incest lobby to champion the right of children to engage in sexual activities with adults of their choice (DeMott 1980). Some investigators describe the gradual induction of "cooperative victims" into sexual relationships which provide "attention" and "nurturance" (Henderson 1983; Krieger et al. 1980). Some of these clinicians seem to assume that if trauma is present, it must be an inherent property of the sexual act itself (Bender and Blau 1937; Yorokoglu 1966). In some cases this is, in fact, the child's view. However, Freud (1896), and later Ferenczi (1949), looked beyond the specifics of the sexual encounter to assess the quality of the victim's overall interpersonal environment. Freud spoke of children's powerlessness in the face of adult demands and their discomfort at having to shift roles from lover to obedient child without explanation. Ferenczi described the "confusion of tongues between adult and child," with the adult's needs, feelings, and perceptions determining the course of the sexual relationship, while the child must suppress his or her true responses.

Psychotherapists regularly encounter patients who describe an incest experience matter-of-factly, sometimes as an aside to a more "important" memory or problem. Such patients may deny that there was any frightening or painful quality in the experience (Barry and Johnson 1958). Of course, this is not an uncommon finding in post-traumatic disorders as well, especially in those cases where dissociation, repression, and other defenses have been exceptionally strong (Horowitz 1976; van der Kolk 1984).

However, the intensity of the traumatic impact of such events must also vary. Freud (1896), and later Rollo May (1975), suspected that psychic pain might actually be less in those cases where the consistent brutality of the perpetrator made the sexual incidents more congruent and expectable for the victim and, thus, less disappointing.

Few psychiatrists would argue about the damaging potential for children who grow up in the most extremely disturbed incest families where a psychotic parent sadistically abuses the children physically and sexually. The hallmarks of this kind of incest include the use of bondage, or burial; the insertion of objects into orifices; the recruitment of other family members as witnesses or co-perpetrators; the involvement of multiple victims, including non–family members, infants, and adults; and the active pursuit of incest pregnancies (Roybal and Goodwin 1982; Goodwin, in press). This is the type of incest most commonly found in the childhood histories of patients with multiple personality disorder (Wilbur 1984), 70 percent of whom are incest victims (Putnam 1984).

However, the circumstances of even these most-damaged families may not meet the strict criteria for childhood trauma that are being developed as post-traumatic disorders begin to be defined in young children (Terr 1983). Incest victims cannot be said to be free of symptoms due to deprivation and pathologic family interaction. They have not been exposed to a single, discrete, overwhelming incident, but to hundreds of assaults, spanning years and developmental phases, and to the concealment, lack of empathy or protection, and hypocrisy that fill the interstices between assaults (Summit 1983; also see Chapter 7).

Nevertheless, contaminated as this system may be with confounding variables, it is no more confounded than the World War I trenches that gave us the patients whose symptoms were first called post-traumatic (Kardiner 1941). Here, too, one found multiple assaults on the self, some more disorganizing than others. Here, too, the shape of the ultimate disorganization was profoundly influenced by the deprivations and distortions learned in the "combat family" (and by those experienced earlier in the patient's own family).

One of the most interesting definitions of trauma is the pragmatic one developed by Richard Kluft (1984b), based on his treatment of over 70 patients with multiple personality disorder. As mentioned above, this disorder is particularly relevant to the problem of incest. Multiple personality disorder is also relevant to the problem of post-traumatic syndromes since fugue, amnesia, and other dissociative symptoms sometimes occur in post-traumatic states (Spiegel 1984). The question Kluft asked was, "What kinds of events trigger the creation of new personalities in children who later present with multiple personality disorder?" By analyzing the characteristics of those experiences that triggered dissociative escapes, he generated the following criteria for a traumatic incident: (*a*) the child fears for his or her own life, (*b*) the child fears that an important attachment figure will die, (*c*) the child's physical intactness and/or clarity of consciousness is breached or impaired, (*d*) the child is isolated with these fears, and (*e*) the child is systematically misinformed, or "brainwashed," about his or her situation. Again, these criteria are not so distant from data collected from Viet Nam veterans, which indicate that symptom severity is influenced by (*a*) exposure to life-threatening combat, (*b*) loss of comrades, (*c*) wounds, illness, and drug use, (*d*) absence of permission to discuss the trauma, and (*e*) participation in atrocities or other activities that require concealment or lead to moral dilemmas (van der Kolk 1984).

Using this pragmatic definition of trauma, one finds that it predicts many of the factors that have been associated with poor prognosis in incest victims. The perpetrator's use of physical force, death threats to the child or to other family members, the child's fears about his or her own physical sensations, the absence of any mirroring or comforting parent figure, the confusing quality of the rationalizations or paranoid thinking used by some families—all of these increase the traumatic potential of the incest experience.

ARE INCEST VICTIMS SYMPTOMATIC?

In 1980, Mrazek and Mrazek reviewed all published reports describing child and adolescent incest victims. Twenty-four publications reported significant symptoms in victims; three publications found no negative effects, and two found both symptomatic and asymptomatic victims. Symptoms recorded included fears, anxiety, sleep disturbances, depression, low self-esteem, guilt, psychosomatic problems, sexual disorders of all types, and behavioral problems.

Adams-Tucker (1982) found symptoms in 100 percent of 28 child incest victims. Maisch (1973) made at least one psychiatric diagnosis in two-thirds of 70 child victims. Becker and co-workers (1982) reported more frequent and severe orgasmic problems in adolescent incest victims as compared to adolescent rape victims. Meiselman

(1978) found that of adult incest victims in psychiatric treatment, three-quarters complained of sexual dysfunction.

Studies that report a high frequency of symptoms in incest victims can be criticized because populations are selected on the basis of a request for psychiatric help, or because a criminal conviction was obtained in the case (opening the question of traumatization by the criminal justice system). Studies that report no symptoms in incest victims also have methodologic problems. These studies often fail to differentiate victims of peer and stranger contacts from victims of classic incest (Renshaw 1982). Some of these studies also fail to include measures that would register post-traumatic symptoms (Burton 1968).

Overall, the symptoms found in incest victims resemble those found acutely in rape victims. Fear, sleep and eating disturbances, guilt, decreased functioning, sexual problems, and irritability—all are found in the rape-trauma syndrome as described by Burgess and Holmstrom (1979). Symptoms in incest victims may be more numerous, more severe, and longer lasting, but this parallels the observation that incest victims have undergone more-numerous sexual assaults over a more-prolonged period. These rape-trauma symptoms, so frequently described for incest victims have been incorporated into checklists for pediatricians who provide forensic pelvic examinations for child victims (National Center on Child Abuse and Neglect 1980). In some jurisdictions the presence of these behavioral symptoms can be used as evidence that the child was sexually abused (National Legal Resource Center 1982). Thus, the legal system appears ready to acknowledge that some child incest victims suffer symptoms of the type found in acute post-traumatic disorders.

RECOGNIZING POST-TRAUMATIC DISORDERS IN INCEST VICTIMS

In the following case examples, victims were found to be symptomatic in the five areas described by Kardiner in his original descriptions of shell-shocked combat veterans. These patients presented with symptoms of (*a*) fear, startle reactions, and anxiety; (*b*) repetition, reenactment, or flashback to the trauma; (*c*) sleep disturbance and other depressive phenomena, including excessive guilt; (*d*) ego constriction or regression; and (*e*) explosive and maladaptive expressions of anger. This symptom list, adapted from Kardiner, overlaps the diagnostic criteria for post-traumatic stress disorder in the *Diagnostic and Statistical Manual of Mental Disorders* (American Psychiatric Association 1980).

The first case describes a very young child. However, the classic nature of her symptoms becomes apparent despite her young age. As treatment has become more available, the average age of incest victims has declined (Goodwin and Geil 1982). If victims of one-time-only sexual abuses are ever to be studied, those subjects will probably come from this preschool-age group, as latency-age victims are likely to have undergone protracted and repeated abuses before they are identified.

> Karen, an only child, age two and one-half, was brought to a pediatrician by her parents after a week-long visit from her maternal grandparents. Karen had brought a knitting needle to her mother, saying, "That belongs to granny and grandpa; they stuck it in my bottom." She also said that her granny had slapped her across the face. Physical findings were consistent with her complaints. In the first two and one-half weeks after the examination, Karen refused to sleep in her own bed, complaining of ghosts in her room. She appeared fearful around men and would plead, "Please don't stick your fingers in my bottom." She had two or three awakenings each night and complained of nightmares in which she was forced to shake hands with a witch. She lost toilet training completely for the first few days and afterward continued night-time wetting. In the playroom, Karen held tightly to her mother and begged her to put all the animal and human toys in the trash "so they won't stick me." Later, she was able to throw the grandparent puppets onto the floor repeatedly. In subsequent sessions she made a "jar full of fire" and jailed the grandparent puppets there. In the second session, Karen described an imaginary playmate named *Married* (sic) who was not afraid of the animals or the grandparents. Karen explained that Married was older and liked to play with snakes. A chair had to be provided for Married at most family functions and whenever the grandparents were spoken of in the play sessions. When we discussed the possible need for Karen to talk to a judge about the "strange things" her grandparents did, Karen said that Married would not be afraid to do that. By the third session all initial symptoms had disappeared. Karen was able to explore the playroom alone with great freedom, although she still kept the grandparent puppets "in jail." We talked about how Married was like a part of her that was still brave even when Karen was most afraid. Married had disappeared by the fifth session. After 18 months, Karen is asymptomatic. Her mother, who recalled her own sexual abuse for the first time during Karen's evaluation, remains in treatment.

Karen's use of an imaginary playmate to deal with the sexual abuse may be a model for the process that leads, in more severe and protracted cases, to the development of multiple personality disorder (Fagan and MacMahon 1984). The child's rapid improvement seems characteristic of the response of such children to adequate protection and the direct interpretation of their dissociative defenses (Kluft 1984a).

The next case illustrates how Kardiner's five symptom clusters are manifested in a victim of late-latency age, and later in the same child during mid-adolescence. On follow-up the now-adolescent victim might be misdiagnosed as having a conduct disorder. Only the interviewer's awareness of the history of family violence makes visible the fear that underlies the adolescent's symptoms.

Jessie was a 12-year-old whose mother had watched while her adoptive father engaged Jessie in finger-penetration and mutual oral sex. The sexual contact had lasted 3 years. Several of Jessie's friends had been genitally fondled by the father. What Jessie had hated most about the abuse were her preorgasmic feelings during cunnilingus. The marriage was violent and the mother had entered battered-women's shelters several times. The family had last been reunited after the father had kidnapped Jessie's 1-year-old brother from a cousin's home in another state. Jessie believed that her brother, too, had been sexually abused. On first interview, Jessie was afraid either to enter the office or to take a walk. She was convinced that her father, because of his criminal connections, would find her and have her killed before his trial, no matter where she was. Jessie's fears were based on her adoptive father's actual threats and on family lore. One of the father's sibs had been executed in a car bombing; Jessie had heard that her father had murdered a colleague several years before. She was adamant that agencies would be unable to protect her, and the history bore this out. Jessie slept restlessly with many awakenings. She usually cried out in her sleep, but recalled no dreams. In waking hours, she often found herself weeping "for no reason." She kept constantly on the alert for vehicles belonging to her father or any of his numerous family. When she believed she saw one of these, she fled to her room and might not leave it for days. Schoolwork suffered because she was often too fearful to attend classes. Her father had kidnapped her from school in the past. She felt hopeless about learning history and science because she "could not think" about those subjects. She lost her temper frequently, and felt "crazy" when she found herself engrossed in complex fantasies about killing her father.

Largely because of family chaos, follow-up was intermittent, until 2 years later, when Jessie was 14. Her mother had contracted a new alliance, with a man who battered her and emotionally abused the children. Jessie had run away from home five times, never succeeding in finding a safer place. She was on probation for stealing blankets and clothes during a runaway on a winter night. She continued to feel it was only a matter of time before her adoptive father found her and killed her. She doubted she would live to adulthood. She was in the process of repeating her eighth-grade year at school; truancy had become an insuperable problem. She had resolved never to let a man touch her, and felt most comfortable with a Lesbian friend. Jessie had male friends, however, including a distributor of pornographic films, who had promised to make her a star. She currently had several broken ribs from "a fight with some girls." She said she was better at fighting than she had been; "my soul just leaves my body; I don't even remember what happened."

In contrast to the first case, this history illustrates what happens to a victim's symptoms in the absence of adequate protection. Despite developmental transformations, symptoms persist. As seen in this patient's use of dissociation, a particular symptom may become identified as a helpful and necessary ally, thus further complicating the task of treatment.

Delayed and chronic post-traumatic symptoms have been best described in adult incest victims (Gelinas 1983). The symptom complex is usually present when the adult seeks treatment during a crisis. Also, symptoms can sometimes be traced back to manifestations during childhood when the pattern may have been quite similar to that already described for child and adolescent victims (Goodwin and Owen 1982). Like child victims, adult victims may have concerns about parents, and about other victims within the family, and may need referral to a child-protection agency to halt the abuse of child relatives (MacFarlane and Korbin 1983; Goodwin et al. 1983).

Mary, a 28-year-old married secretary with one child, came to a crisis clinic with concerns about her sanity. She had just come home from the grocery store and thrown all the groceries on the kitchen floor. She had been reading a book of reminiscences by incest survivors for the past two days and had been unable to sleep. Mary could not recall any time in her life when she had felt relaxed, but the tension of the past 48 hours had been unbearable. The book had reawakened feelings of rage, guilt, and grief about her incest experiences with her father from ages 4 to 12. A few weeks previously, her father had been diagnosed as having dementia. Mary felt trapped and unable to respect herself. She was unsure if she had successfully protected her son from her father's sexual advances. Mary forced herself to participate in marital sexuality, although flashbacks to the incest blocked both arousal and orgasm. Her childhood had been complicated by her mother's psychosis, as well as by her father's sexual abuse of all siblings. Of Mary's five siblings, one had been convicted for pedophilia, one had been diagnosed as schizophrenic, one was alcoholic, one had numerous suicide attempts, and one was a psychotherapist. Mary had been taken to psychiatrists twice in childhood. At age 6, her teacher reported that Mary looked frightened, cried often, was afraid to go to the bathroom, and did not socialize with other children. Tranquilizers were prescribed. At 15, Mary was brought to a guidance clinic by her mother because of runaways, drug use, promiscuity, and chronic rule breaking. She was diagnosed as having a conduct disorder and no further treatment was recommended. Prior incest was not uncovered at either evaluation, even though it was Mary's complaint to her mother about her father's sexual abuse that precipitated the second evaluation.

It should be noted that the diagnoses made when Mary presented as an adult were: dependent personality disorder and marital problems. Her tension, her sleep difficulties, her flashbacks, her inability to cope with sexuality, her unintegrated feelings of rage were still not recognized as the primary symptom complex. However, when brief treatment that focused on reexperiencing the incest trauma was provided, these problems resolved.

CONCLUSION

Most incest experiences can be defined as potentially traumatic. The persistence of professional debate on this issue probably stems from the reluctance of both therapists and victims to explore in detail the day-to-day childhood realities of the incest predicament (Benedek 1984). Fears and threats of death, fears for loved ones, fears about bodily damage, isolation, and misinformation enhance the traumatogenic potential of incest experiences. Most studies report that incest victims develop symptoms. These symptoms are similar to those described in the rape-trauma syndrome, but may be longer lasting and more severe.

Post-traumatic syndromes can be recognized in incest victims, from preschool age to adulthood. They are easily overlooked, however, especially if the interviewer has failed to ask about child abuse and family violence. Therapists may be best advised to refrain from diagnosing personality disorders until post-traumatic symptoms have cleared. Dissociative disorders are the most likely secondary diagnoses. Monitoring the intensity of post-traumatic symptoms is a sensitive way to identify failures in environmental protection, since fear, often unconsciously perceived, is a common trigger for the recurrence of this syndrome.

REFERENCES

Adams-Tucker C: Proximate effects of sexual abuse in childhood: a report on 28 children. Am J Psychiatry 139:1251–1256, 1982

American Psychiatric Association: Diagnostic and Statistical Manual of Mental Disorders, 3rd ed. Washington, DC, American Psychiatric Association, 1980

Balmary M: Psychoanalyzing Psychoanalysis: Freud and the Hidden Fault of the Father. Baltimore, Johns Hopkins University Press, 1982

Barry MJ, Johnson A: The incest barrier. Psychoanal Q 27:485–500, 1958

Becker J, Skinner L, Abel G, et al: Incidence and types of sexual dysfunctions in rape and incest victims. J Sex Marital Ther 8:65–74, 1982

Bender L, Blau A: The reaction of children to sexual relations with adults. Am J Orthopsychiatry 7:500–518, 1937

Benedek E: The silent scream: countertransference reactions to victims. American Journal of Social Psychiatry 4:49–52, 1984

Burgess AW, Holmstrom LL: Rape, Crisis, and Recovery. Bowie, Md, Robert J Brady Co, 1979

Burton L: Vulnerable Children. London, Routledge & Kegan Paul, 1968

DeMott B: The pro-incest lobby. Psychology Today 3:11–16, 1980

Erikson E: Reality and actuality: an address. J Am Psychoanal Assoc 10:451–474, 1962

Fagan J, MacMahon PP: Incipient multiple personality in children: four cases. J Nerv Ment Dis 172:26–36, 1984

Ferenczi S: Confusion of tongues between adults and the child. Int J Psychoanal 30:225–230, 1949

Freud S: The aetiology of hysteria (1896), in The Standard Edition of the Complete Psychological Works, vol. 3. Translated and edited by Strachey J. London, Hogarth, 1962

Freud S: Fragment of an analysis of a case of hysteria (1901, 1905), in The Standard Edition of the Complete Psychological Works, vol. 7. Translated and edited by Strachey J. London, Hogarth, 1953

Freud S: The Origins of Psychoanalysis: Letters to Wilhelm Fliess, Drafts and Notes, 1887–1902. Edited by Bonaparte M, Freud A, Kris E. New York, Basic Books, 1954

Gelinas D: The persisting negative effects of incest. Psychiatry 46:312–332, 1983

Goodwin J: Helping the child who reports incest: a case review, in Sexual Abuse: Incest Victims and Their Families. Edited by Goodwin J. Boston, John Wright/PSG, 1982

Goodwin J: Persecution and grandiosity in incest fathers, in Proceedings of the Seventh World Congress of Psychiatry (in press)

Goodwin J. Geil C: Why physicians should report child abuse: the example of sexual abuse, in Sexual Abuse: Incest Victims and Their Families. Edited by Goodwin J. Boston, John Wright/PSG, 1982

Goodwin J, Owen J: Incest from infancy to adulthood: a developmental approach to victims and families, in Sexual Abuse: Incest Victims and Their Families. Edited by Goodwin J. Boston, John Wright/PSG, 1982

Goodwin J, Sahd D, Rada R: Incest hoax: false accusations, false denials. Bull Am Acad Psychiatry Law 6:269–276, 1979

Goodwin J, McCarty T, DiVasto P: Prior incest in abusive mothers. Child Abuse Negl 5:1–9, 1981

Goodwin J, Cormier L, Owen J: Grandfather–granddaughter incest: a tri-generational view. Child Abuse Negl 7:163–170, 1983

Henderson DJ: Incest, in Comprehensive Textbook of Psychiatry. Edited by Freedman AM, Kaplan HI, Sadock BJ. Baltimore, Williams & Wilkins, 1975

Henderson J: Is incest harmful? Can J Psychiatry 28:34–40, 1983

Horowitz MJ: Stress-Response Syndromes. New York, Jason Aronson, 1976

Kardiner A: The traumatic neuroses of war, in American Handbook of Psychiatry, vol. 1. Edited by Arieti S. New York, Basic Books, 1941

Kluft R: Multiple personality in childhood. Psychiatr Clin North Am 7:121–134, 1984a

Kluft R: Treatment of multiple personality disorder: a study of 33 cases. Psychiatr Clin North Am 7:9–30, 1984b

Krieger MJ, Rosenfeld AA, Gordon A, et al: Problems in the psychotherapy of children with histories of incest. Am J Psychother 34:81–88, 1980

McFarlane K, Korbin J: Confronting the incest secret long after the fact: a family study of multiple victimization with strategies for intervention. Child Abuse Negl 7:225–240, 1983

Maisch H: Incest. London, Andre Deutsch, 1973

Masson JM: The Assault on Truth: Freud's Suppression of the Seduction Theory. New York, Farrar, Straus and Giroux, 1984

May R: The Courage to Create. New York, WW Norton & Co, 1975

Meiselman K: Incest. San Francisco, Jossey-Bass, 1978

Miller A: Thou Shalt Not Be Aware: Society's Betrayal of the Child. New York, Farrar, Straus and Giroux, 1984

Mrazek PB, Mrazek DA: The effects of child sexual abuse: methodological considerations, in Sexually Abused Children and Their Families. Edited by Mrazek PB, Kempe CH. New York, Pergamon Press, 1980

National Center on Child Abuse and Neglect: Sexual abuse of children: Selected readings. Washington, DC, US Department of Health and Human Services, 1980

National Legal Resource Center for Child Advocacy and Protection: Recommendations for improving legal intervention in sexual-abuse cases. Washington, DC, American Bar Association, 1982

Putnam F: The psychophysiologic investigation of multiple personality disorder. Psychiatr Clin North Am 7:31–40, 1984

Renshaw D: Incest: Understanding and Treatment. Boston, Little, Brown and Co, 1982

Roybal L, Goodwin J: The incest pregnancy, in Sexual Abuse: Incest Victims and Their Families. Edited by Goodwin J. Boston, John Wright/PSG, 1982

Spiegel D: Multiple personality as a post-traumatic stress disorder. Psychiatr Clin North Am 7:101–110, 1984

Summit R: The child sexual abuse accommodation syndrome. Child Abuse Negl 7:177–193, 1983

Terr L: Chowchilla revisited: the effects of psychic trauma four years after a school-bus kidnapping. Am J Psychiatry 140:1543–1550, 1983

van der Kolk BA: Post-Traumatic Stress Disorders: Psychological and Biological Sequelae. Washington, DC, American Psychiatric Press, 1984

Wilbur C: Multiple personality and child abuse. Psychiatr Clin North Am 7:3–8, 1984

Yorokoglu A, Kemph JP: Children not severely damaged by incest with a parent. J Am Acad Child Psychiatry 5:111–124, 1966

Chapter 9

Interaction of Trauma and Grief in Childhood

Spencer Eth, M.D.
Robert S. Pynoos, M.D., M.P.H.

Chapter 9

Interaction of Trauma and Grief in Childhood

The interplay of trauma and grief in childhood is a long-neg-lected area of psychiatric concern. This is surprising, given the historic interest in the grief process (Miller 1971; Gardner 1981) and the growing appreciation of the significance of psychic trauma (Terr 1984; Eth and Pynoos 1985). Part of the explanation for this oversight is confusion over the independence of these two clinical phenomena. Some have observed that a parent's death during child-hood is, per se, a psychic trauma. For instance Krueger (1983, 582) comments that: "The real rather than the symbolic or fantasized loss of a parent during development imposes an actual trauma, with implications for intrapsychic organization during development." For Worden (1982, 102), "The loss of a parent through death is obviously a trauma." Similarly, Black (1978), in her review of the literature on the bereaved child, concludes that a parent's death usually constitutes a massive psychic trauma because an immature ego cannot sustain the grief process without suffering injury. As a result, she does not distinguish among modes of death except to suggest that parental suicide is associated with a worse outcome for the child. However, the child observing a sudden murder is in a very different predicament from the child whose parent dies in a hospital from a chronic illness. From our general work with grief-stricken children and, specifically, from our large study of children who have witnessed a parent's homicide, we have been able to isolate the central role of psychic trauma in certain cases of childhood mourning (Pynoos and Eth 1984; Chapter 2). By so doing, we have further clarified the critical processes of trauma mastery and grief resolution in children.

Many previous accounts of children referred months after a violent parental death have too restrictively focused on the child's expression of grief, and have overlooked the maladaptive trauma-resolution that may have also occurred (e.g., Bergen 1958; Scharl 1961). As Singh and Raphael (1981, 211) have cautioned, "Even when the contri-

171

bution of psychic trauma is dramatic, as in the case of a major rail disaster, it may be overlooked when the focus is exclusively on bereavement counseling." We, therefore, elected to evaluate children as soon as possible after the event, using a specially designed, semi-structured-interview technique (Pynoos and Eth, in press). Our aim was to elicit a full description of the child's subjective experience around the time of the violent death. The interview has three phases. First, we engage the children, by having them draw a picture and tell a story. This projective task provides a link to the child's intrusive concerns over issues of grief and trauma. We explore these issues in depth in the second phase, including attending to the child's perceptual and affective experiences. During the closure phase, we review the child's present and future life plans before terminating the session. Follow-up meetings or referrals for formal psychiatric treatment are arranged as indicated. We have found that a thorough exploration of a traumatic death offers the affected child immediate relief and not further distress.

GRIEF

Much has been written about childhood bereavement, in part because of the frequency of its occurrence. Furman (1974) estimates that 1 child in 20 under the age of 18 years has lost a parent through death. Many additional children suffer the experience of losing a sibling or close relative. Grief is the subjective experience and behavior that occurs after a significant loss, while mourning refers to the process of the attenuation of grief as an adaptation to loss (Horowitz et al. 1981). It is now appreciated that children are capable of a wide range of grief responses, whose expression is influenced by the child's level of development, personality, and cultural milieu. The tasks of mourning in childhood are similar to those for adults. The child must first accept the loss through reality testing and then tolerate the experience of the pain of grief. The child may feel sad, angry, guilty, lonely, tired, confused, preoccupied, and perhaps even ill. The deceased will be remembered, as the child struggles to adjust to the new environment. There follows the slow withdrawal of attachment to the deceased and the increasing availability of psychic energy for forging new or stronger relationships.

Grief-stricken children differ in some respects from their adult counterparts. The capacity of children to sustain sadness or dysphoric affects over time increases with age and ego maturity. Because young children have a short attention span, their sadness or pain may go unnoticed by their adult caretakers. Also, they may not be able to fully participate in the normal adult bereavement rituals.

Further, children seek to maintain the attachment to the lost love object despite their conscious knowledge of the reality of death. The child may therefore embark on a complex series of defensive maneuvers aimed at denying the significance of the loss or the associated affects. A poignant illustration is Freud's (1900) anecdote of a 10-year-old who knew his father was dead but couldn't understand why he didn't come home to supper. This issue will be compounded in the case of a violent homicide, when the police abruptly separate the fatally injured parent from the child. While the parent's body is being transported to a distant hospital or morgue, the child may be left wondering where exactly the parent has been taken and whether death has actually occurred. For example, an 8-year-old thought she overhead someone say that her mother was, "naked in cold storage at the coroner's office." She became angry that no one would allow her to visit and dress her mother in warm clothes. Furman (1974) has also drawn attention to the impact of cognitive confusion about the reality of death on the child's capacity to initiate successful mourning.

Children are subject to the same disturbances of mourning that afflict adults. Pathological grief has been defined as "an intensification of grief to the level where the person is overwhelmed, resorts to maladaptive behavior, or remains interminably in the state of grief without progression of the mourning process toward completion" (Horowitz et al. 1980, 1157). The developmental influence on the expression of pathological grief is illustrated by a follow-up study of 25 children whose fathers were killed in the 1963 Israeli War (Elizur 1982). Throughout the period of three and one-half years, over 40 percent of these children showed clinical evidence of pathological grief, characterized by severe behavior problems and marked impairment in social function.

TRAUMA

The term *trauma* has been commonly used as a synonym for severe stress. However, a more precise definition holds that psychic trauma occurs when an individual is exposed to an overwhelming event resulting in helplessness in the face of intolerable danger, anxiety, and instinctual arousal. We disagree with Waelder's (1967) contention that "sometimes the stimulus is of a kind that all, or almost all, people will consider 'traumatic,' (such as) the loss of a parent." Instead, we concur with Sandler (1967) that, "in the vast majority of cases of death of a parent, a trauma in the strict sense of the definition does not occur." Being informed of a parent's death, although distressing, does not automatically qualify as traumatic.

The witnessing of a relative's murder is always painful, frightening, and universally constitutes a psychic trauma. At the core of the trauma is the continued intrusion in the child's mind of the central action, when the lethal physical harm was inflicted (i.e., the plunge of the knife or blast of a gun). The child undergoes an intense perceptual experience involving all sensory modalities. In addition, the child is aware of autonomic arousal and other bodily sensations. Frequently the child will develop the symptoms of a post-traumatic stress disorder (PTSD), and is plagued by intrusive memories, unconscious reenactments, startle reactions, recurrent nightmares, fears of repeated trauma, and avoidant or other symptomatic behaviors (Terr 1981; see also Chapter 2). Other early responses to psychic trauma involve deleterious effects on the child's cognition (including memory, school performance, and learning), affect, interpersonal relations, impulse control, and vegetative function. Case 1 portrays a school-age child's initial course following exposure to lethal traumatic violence.

Michael I., eight years old, lived with his five- and one-year-old brothers and his natural parents, who were experiencing serious marital discord. Following an angry confrontation between Mr. and Mrs. I. at her boyfriend's home, the father returned to their apartment. In an uncontrollable rage, he proceeded to knife his three sons and then slash his own throat. The five-year-old managed to flee to a neighbor, who summoned the police. The infant was found dead, and the older boys were hospitalized for treatment of their cuts. The father was admitted to the prison ward, where he claimed to have no recollection of his attack.

When first seen in their hospital room, the boys were observed to be sharing one bed and playing closely together. Michael openly displayed his wounds on his back and arms. In a friendly, though forceful and dramatic fashion, he described the violent incident both verbally and in art. He drew a hotel and then pounded the paper, exclaiming, "This is how my father stabbed us!" He did not mention his infant brother's death until explicitly asked. Both children were discharged into their mother's care after five days in the hospital.

The boys attended their brother's funeral, but Michael did not mention it spontaneously in his next session. Instead, Michael dwelled on issues of physical safety. He depicted his new home as having a lock on the door large enough to prevent anyone from entering. In another session, he drew a picture of an apartment building and related in elaborate detail the story of a man who had been killed by some neighbors. Michael's anxiety increased appreciably when he learned that a child had been shot and killed near his schoolyard. Several weeks after the father's attack, Michael was described by his mother as engaging in dangerous, aggressive play, resulting in a number of minor accidents. His sessions centered on themes of violence, and he frequently began sentences with the phrase, "When my father killed me. . . ."

TRAUMATIC GRIEF

Although trauma and grief are profoundly different human experiences, a single event can precipitate both responses. From the case example and other studies, it is apparent that coexisting trauma impairs grief work. Burgess (1975) conceptualizes that victim-oriented thought (the horror over manner of death) interferes with ego-oriented thought (the loss of a family member). We too have found that traumatic anxiety is a priority concern for the ego, compromising its ability to attend to the fantasies of the lost object that are integral to the grief process. Furman (1974, 164) notes: "It sometimes appeared that a patient had difficulty in mourning; closer study revealed that the patient's difficulty lay primarily in coping with his anxieties about the circumstances surrounding the death, which his mind could not master and his environment failed to allay." A possible consequence of the ego's unavailability for effective grief work is an aborted or delayed response. Burgess (1975) presents the case of a 13-year-old whose mourning for her 19-year-old murdered sister was delayed for 6 years until the girl reached the same age as her sister's killing, when the grief was precipitated by an anniversary reaction. We have observed that the child's mourning process extends for months longer than the acute traumatic reaction. Consequently, as the traumatic anxiety diminishes, there may be an intensification of grief. Furthermore, birthdays, holidays, and the anniversary serve as reminders of the parent's absence. Special to these children are their ongoing involvement with the criminal justice system which forces them to think about the parent's traumatic death. Reactivation of grief under these circumstances is often overlooked, despite its implications for the child's performance in criminal proceedings. For example, no one was aware that a 5-year-old boy testifying at the trial of his mother's murderer became flooded with sadness at the mention of her name.

Visual Horror

Other traumatic factors contribute to the disruption of normal bereavement as well. The horrifying sight of the disfiguration of the victim forever haunts the child and is a dreaded reminder of the child's pain. Reminiscing, so essential to the bereavement process, may be drastically inhibited because the intrusive images of the violence interfere with the child's efforts to recollect pleasant memories of earlier parent-child interactions. Wolfenstein (1969) refers to the "terrifying image of the parent's death" causing a fearful avoidance of identification. Furman (1974, 61) has also found that in "several instances children's personalities struggled against their identifications with a dead parent because these identifications with a dead parent because these identifications carried the threat of death itself." To ameliorate this aspect of the trauma, the child may seek a means to resurrect a memory of the parent's physical intactness. The funeral can assume a special importance for these children as it offers the opportunity to reestablish a repaired image of the deceased, while confirming the finality of death. A photograph of the parent can prove enormously comforting to the child for the same reason. The child may need professional assistance to address the visual recollections. In play and fantasy the child may be assisted to "fix up" the parent before approaching the memories of the visual horror. As the child achieves relief from these intrusive images, the child can engage in reminiscing, and the grief process is allowed to proceed.

Guilt

A violent, traumatic death accentuates issues of responsibility, possibly highlighting a child's feelings of guilt. Survivor guilt may represent a conflict over the proper assignment of human acccountability. Children may wish at first to avoid the issue by calling the death an accident, but this provides only superficial relief. Revenge fantasies and fears of counterretaliations by the assailant are often conspicuous when the child can easily assign blame, as for instance when the killer is a stranger. However, preoccupations with these aggressive fantasies can prove debilitating to the child when they persist, recur, or challenge impulse control. In situations of family violence, as in Case 1, the child may be thrown into an intense conflict of loyalty. The child may also feel the need to suppress certain thoughts as unacceptable to other family members. Finally, the child will scrutinize his or her own actions during the violent event. The child will commonly formulate a developmentally dependent inner plan of action that, in imagination, could have prevented the killing or saved the victim. These conscious fantasies of third-party intervention by self or others represent attempts to offset the traumatic helplessness. Later, the child may be troubled by feelings of self-blame for not having done more.

Ego Constriction

The violent death, resulting in trauma and grief, can cause a profound ego constriction (Pynoos and Eth, in press). The child may shun intense emotion; suffer the loss of the omnipotentiality of youth, causing the narrowing of life choices; and develop cognitive difficulties. School and learning problems derive from the intrusion of memories and associations to the violent event, from the retarding effects of a markedly depressed affect, and from the evolution of a cognitive style of forgetting. There also can be multiple, enduring effects on memory, as priority is given to reworking traumatic recollections at the expense of meeting the challenge of other tasks. In extreme cases of psychic numbing, there can be long-lasting and devastating effects on the developing personality (Lifton 1967).

Stigma

Compounding the child's dilemma, the violent death damages the network of family and social support. Children may be stigmatized by a homicide sensationalized in the media. Shneidman (1981, 350) recognizes that "it is obvious that some deaths are more stigmatizing, or traumatic than others; death by murder, or by the neglect of oneself or some other person, or by suicide. Survivor victims of such deaths are invaded by an unhealthy complex of disturbing emotions: shame, guilt, hatred, perplexity." The family may respond by implicitly prohibiting any reference to the killing, leaving the grief-stricken child entrenched in a forced silence, and exacerbating the traumatic sequelae (Lister 1982). We have observed that certain families will even avoid reunions during holiday seasons, particularly if associated with the anniversary of the violent death. If they do gather, there is the absence of reminiscing. In fact, spontaneous mention of the deceased by a child is unwelcomed by the adults and usually ignored. If the child feels in constant danger, there may be insufficient emotional strength to mourn properly. A seven-year-old saw his father stabbed to death by a stranger, who was never apprehended. As an adolescent, the boy had no time to grieve, for he was always too busy seeking to protect himself by avenging his father's murder. Whenever spousal or single-parent homicide occurs, the functionally orphaned child requires immediate placement and adaptation to a new home, neighborhood, and school. It is only after the child gains some relief from the traumatic symptoms that he or she can participate actively in the critical decisions affecting life circumstances. In the rare instance where the social nexus is compassionately understanding, the child's ego restitution following traumatic loss can be consolidated, expanded, and even offered as a model to other family and community members.

Reunion Fantasies

Reunion and restitution fantasies are common in bereavement in all ages. For traumatized, grief-stricken children the reunion fantasy not only serves to recapture the lost parent, but also reverses the violence associated with the death. A 4-year-old witnessed her mother shot to death at close range. She drew a picture and told the story of a snowman who melted down each day, but was completely restored by the next morning. Another 11-year-old, whose mother was murdered, felt her mother watching over her from heaven. She believed that her mother would find the killer and tell her, so that she could then notify the police. In addition to evoking the security of her mother's reassuring presence, this girl also employed her fantasy as a means to gain justifiable revenge against the uncaptured assailant. It is that image of violence which can intensify the depressive affect of grief and the helplessness of trauma. As one child lamented, "I couldn't stand it, the way she died." Although a full-blown, major depression is an unusual response, children will experience a serious loss of self-esteem and intense sadness. In that state, suicidal ideation can emerge. Nagera (1970) described a 5½-year-old who reacted like a traumatized child to his mother's death. The child stated, "I'll commit suicide by locking myself in the car and suffocating. I'll be buried next to her." Depression, combined with a reunion fantasy, produced a powerful urge to join the mother's death. Many of the clinical issues precipitated by traumatic grief are illustrated in Case 2.

> The entire C. family, 10-year-old Jane, 7-year-old Al, and their mother and father, were attacked by two men in the family's store. Mr. and Mrs. C. were beaten and then shot to death, execution-style. The children sustained numerous minor injuries to their head and arms. Fortunately, both Jane and Al were able to escape to the street, thereby saving their lives. The children were placed in protective custody by the police, as they were the sole witnesses to the unsolved crime. They were allowed to attend their parents' funerals, but were then returned to custody.
>
> During the first two weeks after the event, Jane spoke of her fear of another attack and her preference to sleep away from the window. When interviewed at three weeks, she seemed composed and pleasant, and was described as behaving like a model child. However, with encouragement, she shared her memories of the crime and how she knew her parents were dead before being told so by the police. She ruminated that she should not have run away from her parents. Instead, she could have died with them. She described terrifying nightmares of the bloody murders and of another attack: "The men will come here and hit me hard on my head and kill me." The more she spoke, the more depressed her thoughts became. Finally she proclaimed, "Nothing would help me feel better. I just want to be dead." She actively imagined killing herself in any way

possible and reuniting with her parents in heaven. These statements were made in a matter-of-fact tone of voice.

DISCUSSION

Children are particularly vulnerable to the additive demands of trauma mastery and grief work. The obligatory efforts at relieving traumatic anxiety can complicate the mourning process, and greatly increase the likelihood of a pathological grief response. There are several case histories in the literature that are suggestive of this interaction of grief and trauma, but that fail to make explicit its significance (e.g., Bowlby 1963) or present confusing formulations. Anderson (1949) clearly describes cases of traumatic grief, including that of an adolescent who was present when his father was killed in a rocket attack, and who subsequently made a suicide attempt. Although the phenomenology is comparable to our Case 2, his theoretical framework is fundamentally different. Anderson views traumatic grief as a single entity presenting with a panoply of features, rather than the superimposition of two separate processes. Thus, Anderson reduces the cause of the adolescent's psychopathology to "his instinctual drives, aggressive and libidinal (which) were the rocket that destroyed his father" (p. 53). Volkan (1970) wrote of an adolescent whose brother was killed in a drugstore while the boys were joking with other teenagers. In fact, each one of Volkan's series of 23 patients suffering from pathological grief reactions had suddenly experienced the death of the "loved–hated one" (p. 232). Levinson (1972, 160) alludes to the role of trauma when he states that: "The time factor is of critical importance in mourning if the bereaved person is not to be overwhelmed by too much anxiety, pain, and depression." However, despite identifying the elements of trauma in sudden death, Levinson explains only that it is the absence of anticipatory mourning that is responsible for the bereavement difficulties.

In the Harvard Bereavement Study of young widows, 24 of 70 respondents had less than two weeks of warning of fatal illness and less than three days notice that death was imminent. Parkes (1975) summarized the findings for the brief-forewarning group: "Sudden and unexpected bereavement constitutes a special risk to psychological and social adjustment. (The) overall picture is of an intense shock reaction rapidly followed by severe separation anxiety and confused feelings of anger and guilt." In a complete account of the study, Parkes and Weiss (1983, 17) speculate that sudden and untimely deaths interfere with the expression of grief and delay its onset, "because of the shock that they produce and the psychological defenses that this evokes." However, sudden and untimely deaths often occur as a result of violence or lethal accidents (Lundin 1984). Unfortunately, Parkes and Weiss did not analyze separately the subgroup who had no warning whatsoever, in order to determine if there were any characteristics of the event that were overwhelming for them. Instead the investigators conclude that bereavement "is the most severe psychological trauma most people will encounter in the course of their lives" (p. ix) and, "even with preparation, there is trauma in loss" (p. 255).

With the onset of the clinical description of post-traumatic stress disorders, it has become important to be more precise in the use of the concept of psychic trauma. We do not disagree with the descriptions of the special psychological risks following sudden or unexpected deaths for either children or adults. We do suggest that, in addition, the circumstances of the death and the degree of exposure of the survivor may directly affect the development of specific post-traumatic symptoms that may alter the course of the grief response. This confusion may reflect an uncritical acceptance of George Engel's (1961) notion that grief for the loss of a loved one is a psychological trauma analogous to physical trauma. If Parkes and Weiss had remained cognizant of the separate contribution of trauma to the phenomenology of grief, some of their data might have been interpreted differently. For instance, they hypothesize that the brief-forewarning widow group tended to avoid visiting the grave as a defense against recognition of reality. Consonant with an appreciation of post-traumatic symptomatology, this behavior may also represent a widow's wish to avoid specific intrusive images and renewed traumatic anxiety from having been present during her spouse's death.

Siggins (1966, 21) recognized that "among the factors contributing to pathological mourning may be the sudden unexpected occurrence of death, or the manner of death itself." It may seem puzzling then that so many authors omit from their case reports "pertinent details regarding the circumstances of the death and reactions to them" (Furman 1974, 246). Freud discussed how a traumatic situation evokes both external and internal dangers. Older psychoanalytic accounts have predominately focused on the intrapsychic conflict aroused by the death, especially the role of preexisting ambivalence toward the deceased, and anger over the loss. The mode of death is peripheral to these intrapsychic issues. Attention to these unconscious elements led Freud (1917) to his classic formulation that internalization of ambivalence toward the lost object is the major cause of morbid grief. Psychoanalytic accounts have not emphasized, in the witnessing of a traumatic death, the psychological sequelae of the traumatic helplessness. There is no doubt about the importance of intrapsychic conflict in the etiology of pathological mourning. We would suggest that, in cases of traumatic witnessing of deaths, these conflicts also interfere with the recovery from post-traumatic symptoms as well.

Many nonanalytic investigators have also neglected to consider whether the manner of death was traumatic for the mourner. This oversight confounds a number of studies of the symptomatology and management of acute grief, where the direct effects of a traumatic event, which may have been associated with the death, go unexamined. Maddison (1968) found that sudden death, or death with minimal warning, of a spouse does not render the survivor more prone to a worse outcome. Clayton (1968) concurred that the duration of the fatal illness is unrelated to the symptomatology of widows and widowers. But a recent study (Lundin 1984) documented that persons exposed to the sudden and unexpected loss of a close relative are subject to increased morbidity and should be regarded as a high-risk group. All of these studies fail to address the relative contribution of the two co-variables, the suddenness of the death and its traumatic nature. The subjects were not examined for the presence of specific post-traumatic stress disorder symptomatology in light of the circumstances of the death and their degree of exposure. Likewise, an otherwise well-designed study of the association between early parental loss and later mental illness neglects the possible traumatic component of childhood grief (Pfohl 1983) by omitting reference to the modes of death, the exposure of the child, and the children's particular responses at the time.

Treatment Issues

So far, we have stressed the independence of trauma and grief and underscored their clinical differences. However, these two processes share certain salient features in common. Traumatized and grief-stricken parents are plagued by intrusive thoughts, painful affects, and fears of being overwhelmed. There are consequent efforts to avoid reminders of the trauma of the deceased, feelings of hopelessness over the irreversibility of the event, and a sense of personal guilt for having failed to do more. Both processes place enormous demands on psychic energy, which would otherwise be channeled into new relationships or challenges. The courses of trauma and grief are comparable as well. The natural histories are characterized by an abrupt onset after the psychosocial stressor, followed by an acute phase, and then a slow recovery with periodic reactivations, such as anniversary responses. For both syndromes there are a variety of mediating factors, including the presence of supportive objects, which can affect outcome. And importantly traumatized and grief-stricken patients are responsive to focal, brief psychotherapy. In fact, these similarities may have contributed to disguising the elements of trauma in certain cases of grief. Although these two processes may overlap, each has its own burdensome psychic agenda and must be attended to uniquely.

We believe that an early treatment focus on psychic trauma will have a beneficial effect on the child's mourning and on the overall outcome. Traumatic memories are intrusive and ego-dystonic and can be readily addressed in session. For example, Zeanah and Burk (1984) described the treatment of a four-year-old who was first seen one month after watching her father strangle her mother to death: "All of her symptoms seemed to be responses to and expressions of extreme anxiety," warranting the diagnosis of post-traumatic stress disorder. A prompt, complete exploration offers relief and facilitates trauma mastery. We therefore disagree with Lehrman (1956), who cautions that "treatment should proceed slowly" in case of untimely death. That deliberate, conservative approach is often out of synchrony with the child's own attempt to resolve the traumatic crisis.

Following an alleviation of the traumatic anxiety, the child will be able to cope with grief work unencumbered by contamination with traumatic issues. This may allow for the unfolding of the mourning process and its associated affects in those children stymied by aborted grief. Treatment experiences with the survivors of the 1977 Beverly Hills Supper Club fire confirm the applicability of these principles to work with traumatic grief in adults:

> In cases where both intrapsychic trauma and loss were present, the psychotherapy seemed to proceed spontaneously in a sequential manner, namely, working through with regard to trauma including the overwhelming anxiety of death, feelings of helplessness, shame, as well as defenses protecting against these strong affects came first. When they were sufficiently dealt with . . . , a spontaneous progression seemed to ensue in which the patient was able to take on the as yet not worked-through aspects of grief relating to losses in his experience (Lindy 1983, 608).

We, too, have been impressed that after proper attention is paid to the traumatic elements, many children will then exhibit a spontaneous progression to open expressions of grief. Children who had previously shown no signs of grief will suddenly begin to cry over the loss, to reminisce with warmth and sadness over memories of the deceased, and to directly seek comfort and aid in addressing the reality of the death and the life changes that have resulted.

An arrest of normal mourning may occur when insufficient therapeutic attention is paid to relieving traumatic anxiety. The consequences of the resulting aborted grief may not be fully evident for many years, perhaps not until the grief is reactivated in adulthood. Levinson (1972) provides a compelling account of a psychiatric resident whose patient died suddenly of a myocardial infarction, leaving a young son. The therapist had experienced his own father's death as a child under similar circumstances and had not worked through the loss. After several days of severe anxiety and self-reproach, the resident left his program in mid-year and secured a research fellowship without any clinical responsibilities. Residues of traumatic grief can also be appreciated in tales of the occult. Anna Freud (1967) speculated that "lost souls" searching for former loved ones function as a derivative of longing projected into the image of a lost object. We wonder whether haunted houses, ghosts, and changelings represent reifications of the objects of traumatic grief.

In children suffering from pathological grief taking the form of suicidality, therapeutic attention directed toward the traumatic helplessness and passivity can diminish guilt. The child is encouraged to assume an active role in confronting the traumatic situation in session, and thereby recognizes the reality limitations on what could have been done at the time of the violent death. As those experiences are worked through, the child can be supported in reconciling any ambivalence toward the lost object.

CONCLUSION

Although bereavement following violent death will inevitably prove more difficult, it need not defeat the patient's efforts at recovery. The dual tasks of trauma mastery and grief resolution are crucial, and therapeutic work can succeed when both are addressed. We must not allow the disabling legacy of traumatic grief to last a lifetime.

REFERENCES

Anderson C: Aspects of pathological grief and mourning. Int J Psychoanal 30:48–55, 1949

Bergen ME: The effects of severe trauma on a four-year-old child. Psychoanal Study Child 13:407–429, 1958

Black D: Bereaved child. J Child Psychol Psychiatry 19:287–292, 1978

Bowlby J: Pathological mourning and childhood mourning. J Am Psychoanal Assoc 11:500–541, 1963

Burgess AW: Family reaction to homicide. Am J Orthopsychiatry 45:391–398, 1975

Clayton P, Desmarais L, Winokur G: A study of normal bereavement. Am J Psychiatry 125:169–178, 1968

Elizur E, Kaffman M: Children's bereavement reactions following death of the father: II. J Am Acad Child Psychiatry 21:474–480, 1982

Engel GL: Is grief a disease? Psychosom Med 23:18–22, 1961

Eth S, Pynoos R: Developmental aspects of psychic trauma, in Trauma and Its Wake. Edited by Figley CR. New York, Brunner/Mazel, 1985

Freud A: About losing and being lost. Psychoanal Study Child 22:9–19, 1967

Freud S: Interpretation of dreams (Chapter 5, footnote 1909), (1900), in The Standard Edition of the Complete Psychological Works of Sigmund Freud, vol. 4. Edited by Strachey J. London, Hogarth Press, 1953

Freud S: Mourning and melancholia (1917), in The Standard Edition of the Complete Psychological Works of Sigmund Freud, vol. 14. Edited by Strachey J. London, Hogarth Press, 1957

Furman E: A Child's Parent Dies. New Haven, Yale University Press, 1974

Gardner RA: Death of a parent, in Basic Handbook of Child Psychiatry, vol. 4. Edited by Noshpitz JD. New York, Basic Books, 1981

Horowitz MJ, Wilner N, Marmar C, et al: Pathological grief and the activation of latent self-images. Am J Psychiatry 137:1157–1162, 1980

Horowitz MJ, Krupnick J, Kaltreider N, et al: Initial psychological response to parental death. Arch Gen Psychiatry 137:316–323, 1981

Kahn L: No Time to Mourn. Vancouver, Laurelton, 1978

Krueger DW: Childhood parent loss: developmental impact and adult psychopathology. Am J Psychother 37:582–592, 1983

Lehrman SR: Reactions to untimely death. Psychiatr Q 30:564–578, 1956

Levinson P: On sudden death. Psychiatry 35:160–173, 1972

Lifton RJ: Death in Life. New York, Random House, 1967

Lindy JD, Green BL, Grace M, et al: Psychotherapy with survivors of the Beverly Hills Supper Club fire. Am J Psychother 37:593–610, 1983

Lister ED: Forced silence: a neglected dimension of trauma. Am J Psychiatry 139:872–876, 1982

Lundin T: Morbidity following sudden and unexpected bereavement. Br J Psychiatry 144:84–88, 1984

Maddison D: The relevance of conjugal bereavement for preventive psychiatry. Br J Med Psychol 41:223–233, 1968

Miller JBM: Children's reactions to the death of a parent: a review of the psychoanalytic literature. J Am Psychoanal Assoc 19:697–719, 1971

Nagera, H: Children's reactions to the death of important objects: a developmental approach. Psychoanal Study Child 25:360–400, 1970

Parkes CM: Unexpected and untimely bereavement: a statistical study of young Boston widows and widowers, in Bereavement: Its Psychosocial Aspects. Edited by Schoenberg B, Gerber I, Wiener A, et al. New York, Columbia University Press, 1975

Parkes CM, Weiss RS: Recovery from Bereavement. New York, Basic Books, 1983

Pfohl B, Stangl D, Tsuang MT: The association between early parental loss and diagnosis in the Iowa 500. Arch Gen Psychiatry 40:965–967, 1983

Pynoos R, Eth S: The child as witness to homicide. Journal of Social Issues 40:87–108, 1984

Pynoos R, Eth S: Witness to violence: the child interview. J Am Acad Child Psychiatry (in press)

Sandler J: Trauma, strain, and development, in Psychic Trauma. Edited by Furst SS. New York, Basic Books, 1967

Scharl AH: Regression and restitution in object loss: clinical observations. Psychoanal Study Child 16:471–480, 1961

Shneidman ES: Postvention: the care of the bereaved. Suicide Life Threat Behav 11:349–359, 1981

Siggins LD: Mourning: a critical survey of the literature. Int J Psychoanal 47:14–25, 1966

Singh B, Raphael B: Postdisaster morbidity of the bereaved. J Nerv Ment Dis 169:203–212, 1981

Terr L: Psychic trauma in children: observations following the Chowchilla school-bus kidnapping. Am J Psychiatry 138:14–19, 1981

Terr LC: Children at acute risk: psychic trauma, in Psychiatry Update, vol. 3. Edited by Grinspoon L. Washington, DC, American Psychiatric Press, 1984

Volkan V: Typical findings in pathological grief. Psychiatr Q 44:231–250, 1970

Waelder R: Trauma and the variety of extraordinary challenges, in Psychic Trauma. Edited by Furst SS. New York, Basic Books, 1967

Wolfenstein M: Loss, rage, and repetition. Psychoanal Study Child 24:432–460, 1969

Worden JW: Grief Counseling and Grief Therapy. New York, Springer Publishing, 1982

Zeanah CH, Burk GS: A young child who witnessed her mother's murder: therapeutic and legal considerations. Am J Psychother 38:132–145, 1984